A CHANGE FO

C000138314

A Woman's Guide through the Menopause

PATRICIA DAVIS

A CHANGE FOR THE BETTER

A Woman's Guide through the Menopause

Cartoons by Anne Ward
Index compiled by Lyn Greenwood

SAFFRON WALDEN
THE C.W. DANIEL COMPANY LIMITED

First published in Great Britain in 1993
by The C.W. Daniel Company Limited
1 Church Path, Saffron Walden
Essex, CB10 1JP, England

ISBN 0 85207 265 1

This book is printed on part-recycled paper

Designed by Peter Dolton
Produced by Book Production Consultants plc, Cambridge
Typeset by Cambridge Photosetting Services
and printed by
St Edmundsbury Press Ltd, Bury St Edmunds, Suffolk

THIS BOOK
IS DEDICATED TO
MORAIG MACDONALD

CONTENTS

PART III: A CHANGE FOR THE BETTER

APPENDICES

ACKNOWLEDGEMENTS

I WANT TO thank the following practitioners who read the sections covering the various therapies. Their comments, corrections and additions contributed so much to the chapter "Widening Your Choices": Ursula Athene, homoeopathy; Jitindriya Bell, reflexology; Liz Dolton, healing; Penny Grevatt, Yoga; Martin Muchan, Alexander Technique; Maria Offutt, craniosacral therapy; Jonathan Parker, osteopathy; Sheila Tozer, acupuncture and TCM and Julie Walker, shiatsu.

Thanks also to Angela Chappell in Zimbabwe and Helen Ranger in South Africa for valuable correspondence, to Naomi Hull and members of Stroud U3A for welcoming me into their group, to Helen Pope for pointing me towards some important nutritional information and to Anne Ward for her wonderful cartoons and all the laughs we have shared while planning them.

But, above all, I offer my heartfelt thanks to all the women who have shared their experiences, hopes and fears with me: without them, this book would not have been possible.

How This Book Came To Be

IN THE AUTUMN of 1991 I was teaching a group of women at an aromatherapy workshop a few weeks before my second book ("Subtle Aromatherapy") was published. I also had an exhibition of my paintings opening in two weeks time, and over lunch one of the assistant tutors asked me when the book was due out, and the other asked for the dates of the exhibition. At this, one of the students asked "How on Earth do you manage to do it all – write books, paint pictures AND teach us lot?" I answered, laughing "The menopause is a great thing!". "What do you mean?" she asked, obviously very puzzled, so I explained that when a woman has been menstruating for 30 years or so, maybe with PMS or cramps or backaches each month, or just a day or two when she felt a bit less energetic than usual, and then all that stops, it is like being handed a whole lot of extra time and energy on a silver salver! The student exclaimed "That's the first positive thought about the menopause I've ever been offered!".

The other students joined in and I was shocked to realise that everyone of them had fears and negative expectations of the menopause and the years following it – and these were women studying an alternative therapy, who could be presumed to know more than average about health and the workings of their bodies. As they talked, it became clear that their fears were fed and magnified by much of what they read in books and the press, so I expanded a bit on my original statement, talking about some of the other delights of being an older woman, the honoured place occupied by older women in some societies and what Margaret Mead, the great anthropologist, called "post-menopausal zest".

When the lunch-break came to an end and I called the group back to work, my original questioner said "You've got to write a book about this, you know. You owe it to us."

....

So – here it is! and I hope it will go some way towards dispelling those fears and helping women to experience menopause as a natural transition from one important phase of their life to another, different but equally important.

TOTNES,
Devon,
June 1993.

INTRODUCTION

THE ONE TIME in a woman's life that most closely resembles the menopause is adolescence. Think about the similarities: our hormones behave unpredictably, the shape and function of our bodies change, the whole process may take several years and at the end of it we enter a new phase of our life. And yet adolescence is generally regarded as "a good thing" and menopause is not. Why is this so? Adolescence is associated with "growing up" and menopause with "growing old" and while the majority of young girls want to "grow up" – to become sexually mature women – few women (or men, for that matter) relish the thought of growing old.

Thinking about aging makes us confront the issue of our own death. There may also be fears about illness, disability, loneliness or loss of mental faculties in our latter years. These are things which affect men and women equally, but there are other issues surrounding menopause which give rise to so much anxiety and negativity.

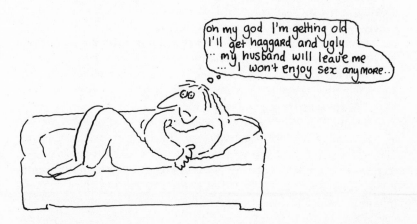

"I'm afraid of losing my looks."

"I'm really scared my husband will leave me for a younger woman."

"I worry about holding on to my job as I get older. There is so much emphasis on youth in my profession (television)."

"I'm afraid I won't enjoy sex after my periods end."

"My mother had a really bad time during the change and I'm afraid I will too, but she won't talk about what she actually means by "a bad time", so I don't really know what to expect."

Knowing what to expect is a first step to dispelling fears, and knowing where to look for help with such problems as do arise is a second. Only about 20% of pre-menopausal women know what to expect in the years ahead, so in this book I have tried to explain clearly what happens to women's bodies in mid-life, the problems they may encounter and many different ways of dealing with them, so that YOU can choose which suits you best.

Talking to women of all ages – those who have completed their menopause and younger women who have not entered it yet, as well as those who are currently passing through it – I realised that a common thread running through many of their concerns was a feeling of helplessness, of absence of choice, a fear of not being in control of their own bodies or emotions.

A frequent worry is that there often seems to be no middle ground between long-term drug taking and resigning oneself to debilitating symptoms and a process of slow, or not-so-slow, physical decline. Many women are – quite rightly – concerned about the side effects and risks involved in many of these drugs. So, in addition to looking at the medical options, I have included information about a variety of alternative/complementary therapies which offer effective ways to combat menopausal discomfort and post-menopausal disease. YOU DO HAVE A CHOICE and it is your right to use it.

I have included many self-help strategies, as well as orthodox and alternative therapies, because knowing what you can do FOR YOURSELF is liberating and empowering.

Quite a few of these self-help methods involve what we eat and how much we use our bodies, in short, those overused words diet and exercise but I beg you to stay with me and not to skip those sections of the book. They are not concerned with yet another slimming regime, nor the latest fad in figure control, but the two most important and effective things you can do to combat menopausal miseries and postmenopausal deterioration of your physical body. (Do you know which foods help slow down aging or what exercise prevents bone disease?) That they **will** help you to go on looking good and feeling good for many decades is just the bonus!

I know that when I read that sort of good advice in a book, there is always the temptation to think "Oh, it's all very well for her to sit there writing that! She's probably as thin as a rake, fabulously beautiful and stinking rich into the bargain!" So I want to tell you that I don't find diet and exercise easy, either. I put weight on easily, and most of my passions are sedentary ones: painting, writing, reading, listening to music. But the research I have done in the process of writing this book has so convinced me of the importance of appropriate exercise and the right foods for older women that I've started following my own good advice.

A large part of the book is concerned with the physical body: the changes that happen in the body, the discomforts, problems or more serious illnesses that may follow these changes, and ways of preventing and treating them. The reason for this is simply that the body is the vehicle through which we experience life. An ailing, aching body is not the best vehicle for setting out on the great adventure which is the second half of your life.

When I say "the second half of your life" I mean that quite literally. If you are a woman in a Western culture and experiencing the menopause now, you are likely to live for another 30 or 40 years, in other words half of an average lifetime, and certainly far more than half of your adult life.

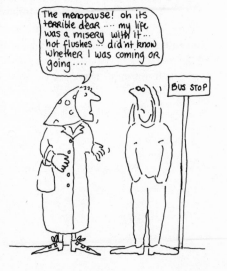

What are you going to do with all those years?

Are you going to live them to the full: working, playing, loving, studying, creating, adventuring and developing as a person, or are you content to settle for a steady decline towards senility and death?

You might not have thought in these terms before,

because the prospect of half a lifetime ahead of you when your child-bearing years have ended is a new one. Even our mothers' generation did not have anything like such a lengthy expectation of life, and if we look back only a couple of hundred years, many women died before ever reaching menopause. Consequently, many of our attitudes towards and expectations of menopause and after are conditioned by the idea that it is the beginning of the end.

If we are going to enjoy our increased lifespan and use it creatively we have to separate the truth about women's lives from the old wives tales, outdated medical myths and social taboos that have surrounded menopause and aging.

My real purpose in writing this book is to share with you the knowledge that menopause is not an end, but a doorway into the next part of your life. I shall be inviting you to look through that doorway at some of the new opportunities that await you and introducing some of the women who have done exciting things in the second half of their lives.

Yes, it involves change, and all change is challenging. Even those changes that we ardently wish for present us with stresses and challenges. Remember your first job, your first love-affair, the first home that was really your own: these were probably changes that you wanted very much but you can almost certainly recall the personal challenges they involved as well. Moving through menopause into the next stage in your life is no different.

Change is much more difficult to cope with when we resist it, pretend it is not happening, try to maintain the status quo. When we embrace change we can make it work for us.

Remember those 30 or 40 years that lie ahead.

This book is about enjoying them.

PART I
WHAT CAN YOU EXPECT?

This part of the book sets out to
explore the simple facts about menopause
and separate them from the myths.

I hope that knowing where some of the
myths come from, what happens during
menopause and how other women have
experienced it will help to demystify the
subject and make it easier for you to
know what is happening or what
is likely to happen to you.

MYTHS, LIES AND
MEDICAL TEXTS

IF THERE IS one single factor that influences our experience of menopause, it is the attitude of the society in which we live. When I talk with young women, I find that their expectation of menopause is almost totally negative. Those in their late thirties and early forties are often very apprehensive, and it is hardly surprising when we consider that they are surrounded by negative messages about middle aged women in general and menopause in particular. Old wives' tales abound and jokes about hot flushes are always an easy way to raise a laugh. (When did you see a SERIOUS play about a menopausal woman and the issues she faces?) Tales and jokes alike are nearly always based on misconceptions about women's lives and bodies.

Many of the fallacies about menopause have their origin in nineteenth century and earlier beliefs about women, which in turn reflect the social climate and medical knowledge of their day. To understand how these affect women at menopause we need first to look at Victorian attitudes to all women.

Central to all of them was the assumption that a woman's primary function is to have babies, her secondary role being as carer and provider of comfort for her husband and his children. ("His" children, you note, not "their" children, for in law the husband had absolute rights over his offspring and their mother had none.) This being so women, except in the very poorest strata of society, were not expected to work outside the home, nor to have any intellectual, artistic or other interests of their own.

In 1852 Florence Nightingale wrote a bitter diatribe against the sterility of women's lives. "Why have women passion, intellect, moral activity – these three – and a place in society where no one of the three can be exercised?" she wrote. By great effort of will, she showed that women could indeed exercise these gifts, and there were other exceptions: the pioneers who founded all-female colleges when the ancient universities were closed to them, the first women medical students, the female art-students who fought for the right to attend life-classes with their male colleagues. Such women, though, were a tiny minority: in general the intellectual or artistic woman has always been a maverick and often viewed as eccentric, scandalous or even

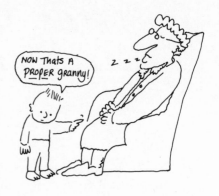

NOW That's A PROPER granny!

z z z

dangerous. In the nineteenth century such women were even imagined to be a danger to themselves! Doctors and the early psychoanalysts thought that too much intellectual activity was bad for women, and those who were not content with a domestic role were often diagnosed as ill. Some of them were, indeed, ill because their restricted lives led to depression and psychosomatic illness.

The effect of this on a woman at mid-life was that when her role as child-bearer came to an end, her life was shorn of its central purpose and little or nothing in her earlier experience prepared her to fill that gap. Even as late as the 1940's a leading psychoanalyst (and a woman, at that) wrote of the "justified grief" of menopausal women as their children grew up, and it is still quite common to ascribe any depression experienced by a woman in her 40's or 50's to the "empty nest syndrome".

Extending from the belief that women's primary, if not only, role was to have babies came the notion that their sexuality was entirely geared to reproduction. Therefore, it followed logically that a woman who was no longer fertile was no longer sexual. Indeed, even women of child-bearing age were not expected to enjoy sex, at least if they were "respectable": this was the age of "lie back and think of England". Menopausal or post-menopausal women who did not suppress their sexuality were subjected to horrendous "medical" treatments, including packing ice into the vagina and applying leeches to the vulva.

Small wonder, then, that menopause became a time to dread, to be spoken of in whispers if at all, and never within earshot of men, or even of younger women.

But why, you may ask, do such negative expectations of menopause still persist when women can be astronauts or prime ministers, climb Everest or sail single-handed round the world? Partly because of that whispering. If women don't talk about menopause, even to each other, the subject acquires the status of a taboo and the most powerful taboos are those that we observe in our families. There are plenty of older women alive whose grandmothers were born during Victoria's reign and not a few whose mothers were. Indeed, there are some grand old ladies in their 90's who were born towards the end of the last century. Two or three generations are not long in the lifetime of a taboo.

To further understand why the old myths die hard, we need to look a bit harder at the idea that women's role is having babies. One of the reasons it persists is that it has a core of truth. Women, and only women, have babies and this fact is deeply rooted in our race-memory, indeed in our genetic memory. Every species must reproduce itself and the impulse to do so is built into our genes. What is

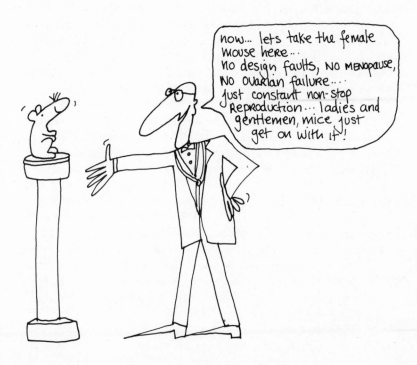

fallacious about the idea is the implication that women CAN'T DO ANYTHING ELSE and that, of course, is where it disempowers older women.

So much focus on fecundity is grotesquely inappropriate now, in a world where overpopulation threatens our very future. When less importance is attached to the ability of young women to reproduce, and more to their other skills and talents, perhaps the transition from youth to maturity will be smoother.

The advent of reliable birth-control in the present century and especially the Pill in the 1960'a freed women from that genetic imperative by allowing them to choose whether or not to have children and if they did want children, to decide when.

The Pill also allowed women to separate their sexuality from childbearing. In effect, they could choose to become temporarily infertile. And yet, the notion persists that women who are no longer fertile have no sexual feelings (or, at least, that they should not). The first women who took the Pill have reached mid-life now, and it may be that they will be the generation who finally kill off the old fictions. A danger which I perceive, though, is that the image of woman-as-mother is being replaced by the image of woman-as-nymphet. Cinema, television, newspapers and magazines bombard us continually with pictures that say "young is desirable, young is available". We have exchanged the madonna for the whore ...or should I say we have exchanged the madonna for Madonna?

The old notion that women only exist to have babies also gave rise to the medical view that the womb and ovaries served no further purpose once a woman had produced a number of children, so hysterectomy was advised for any and every gynaecological problem. We know now how important the ovaries are for a woman's health and well-being in later life, yet some doctors still recommend total hysterectomy when there are less damaging alternatives available.

Even the way doctors write and speak about menopause is full of negative messages. Who wants to be told that she is suffering from "ovarian failure" when her ovaries have simply and naturally reached the end of their egg-producing years? To a doctor, this just means that the ovaries are not making eggs any more, but to a woman on the receiving end it can sound like a value-judgement and "failure" is something about which we often feel guilty.

Worse still are those doctors who really are making value-judgements, such as describing the menopause as "One of Nature's

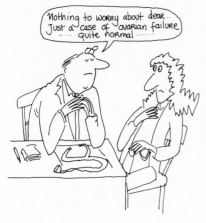

design faults". This phrase was used, very recently, to justify using hormone replacement and implanted donor eggs to enable post-menopausal women to give birth. The implied logic was that other mammals do not have a menopause so there is something wrong with women because they do. Even if we disregard the fact that a baby mouse is mature in a couple of weeks while a human baby needs 18 or more years of nurture, this completely ignores the value to society, and to herself, of the 20 or 30 years that a woman can expect to live after she stops ovulating.

All that I have written so far is true of modern, urbanized society. It is perhaps ironic that to find models of powerful, active women regardless of age, we may need to look back five centuries. Those nineteenth-century attitudes that we still see perpetuated, obscured an earlier culture with a quite different view of women. I have in front of me some pictures from illuminated manuscripts showing mediaeval women at work and play. Here are women gardeners and farmers, builders (yes, really heaving stones and mortar around), miners, millers, midwives, archers, authors, artists, spinners, weavers, wine-makers and musicians. At play, they sing, dance, hunt with falcons, write letters, play chess and pelt men with snowballs! Would you rather have them as role-models or our corsetted, crinolined great-grandmothers?

At the present day, women in non-urbanised societies are more likely to see menopause as a positive time in their life and less likely to suffer physical symptoms than their urbanised sisters. That this is due to their social experiences rather than any ethnic difference is well illustrated in Southern Africa: black women in the rural areas are inclined to see menopause as a welcome relief from constant childbearing. (Family planning is not welcomed by the rural menfolk because the number of children a woman has is seen as proof of her husband's virility.) In many places, post-menopausal women acquire higher status in their villages, but once these people move into the towns, the old beliefs begin to disappear and the women start to experience more physical difficulties at menopause. The emergent black middle class have the same problems as white women.

Perhaps we can learn from the women of non-industrialised societies, whether in mediaeval Europe or rural Africa. Certainly we need to shake off the conditioning of the past 150-200 years, the most insidious aspect of which is that women came to believe the myths themselves. Many, alas, still do.

I hope that by setting out clearly some facts about menopause and about older women's lives I can help to explode some of the fallacies.

2

WHAT CAN I EXPECT?

NOW THAT WE have had a look at some of the myths about menopause, we can start looking at the facts, and the first thing I want to do is to set out clearly what happens to the body at menopause and some of the different ways in which you may experience this.

The word menopause, strictly speaking, means the point at which menstruation stops altogether, but it is most often used to describe the time, ranging from a few months to several years, leading up to this, and it is in this sense that I shall use it throughout this book.

When a baby girl is born, she has in her ovaries hundreds of thousands of rudimentary egg cells but of course she is not yet able to have babies of her own so the eggs do not ripen and leave the ovaries until her body is mature enough to support a pregnancy – at least theoretically. Somewhere in her early or mid teens, the first of these eggs ripen and passes down her fallopian tubes into her womb. At first the release of eggs (ovulation) may not be at all regular, but eventually the process settles down into a cycle lasting on average 28 to 31 days. The lining of the womb changes at the time each egg is released, making it suitable to support and nourish the egg if it is fertilised. If it is not fertilised bleeding happens about two weeks after the egg was released and the pattern of monthly periods is established. For most women, these continue more or less regularly except if they are interrupted by a pregnancy. The whole cycle involves a number of hormones which interact with each other and we'll be looking at these in much more detail later: the role of hormones in our lives is so important that they warrant a whole chapter to themselves. For the moment, it is enough to know that the main female hormone, oestrogen, is made in the ovaries as part of the cycle.

Sometime in the mid-forties (for most women) this process begins to go into reverse: instead of ovulation happening roughly once in every month, it becomes irregular. As a result, the amount of oestrogen circulating in the body drops. There seems to be a kind of "leap-frog" effect: fewer eggs ripening means less oestrogen being produced, but less oestrogen in the body hastens the decline in egg production until ovulations stops altogether. The drop in oestrogen levels is also a major factor that triggers other bodily changes.

The uterus (womb) which is originally about the size of your clenched fist, gradually shrinks until it is about the size of a walnut and its very elastic muscles become rather tough and fibrous. This is because it is no longer stimulated by the flow of hormones from the ovaries to prepare it for an egg.

The drop in oestrogen levels affects the rest of the reproductive system, too. The walls of the vagina very gradually get thinner and less elastic and the glands that produce vaginal lubrication do not work quite so efficiently.

Oestrogen benefits all our muscles, not only those of the reproductive system, also our skin and hair, and as we get older and have less circulating oestrogen, we lose a certain amount of muscle tone and elasticity of the skin.

Oestrogen seems to give women some protection against heart disease, and post-menopausal women are at greater risk of heart attacks than before. The other risk in later years which is also linked to loss of oestrogen is osteoporosis (brittle bones) and because these are both serious topics you'll find them discussed at some length later in the book.

Knowing these facts is, I think, essential but it still doesn't tell you how these things will feel when they happen, how long it all takes, or what problems might arise, so I shall try to answer those questions next.

For the majority of women, the first indication that they are entering the menopause is a change in their pattern of menstruation. Periods may be further apart or closer together or they may stop for several months and then start again. Bleeding may become either lighter or heavier. For example, periods may remain regularly timed, but get gradually more scanty or they may get lighter and further apart. They may come closer together with heavier bleeding, or they may be quite unpredictable with longer and shorter gaps between. All of these patterns are possible and perfectly normal. Eventually periods stop altogether. This may happen quite quickly or it can take several years. For some women, periods simply stop without any warning but that is fairly unusual and for most of us the process of change takes between one and five years.

The first changes in the pattern of regular menstruation may begin at any time between the early and late forties and the average age at which periods end altogether is 51, but this can vary by quite a few years either way and any time between the mid-forties and the mid-fifties can be thought of as normal. About fifty per cent of women stop menstruating by the time they reach 50, and very few will have periods beyond the age of 56. There is no way of predicting the timing of menopause: an early start to menstruation in adolescence does not necessarily mean an early menopause and vice versa. Menopause is usually described as early if all menstruation has stopped by the time a woman is in her early forties, though a very few women (about one in every hundred) stop menstruating in their thirties or even sooner. Nobody knows why, though a great deal of research is being done on this problem currently. One theory (which makes sense in the light of what we do know about menopause) is that the timing is more or less determined before a baby girl is born by the number of rudimentary egg cells developed in the foetus. A baby girl born with significantly fewer egg cells would experience menopause earlier. Certainly nothing in a woman's lifestyle: health, sexual activity or absence of it, or whether or not she has borne children, appear to have any significance with regard to timing.

One aspect of lifestyle that does appear to have an influence is smoking and women who smoke heavily generally have an earlier menopause than others. (If you have had difficult periods, you might think an early menopause is something to be thankful for, but in fact women who stop menstruating early risk more long-term health problems than those who stop later.) There is also an increasing amount of evidence that heavy smokers experience more problems around this time than non-smokers in addition to being at greater risk of strokes, heart attacks and other health problems.

To illustrate some of the different ways in which the end of regular menstruation might be experienced, I will let three women tell their own stories:

Grace is a teacher, in her late fifties who describes her experience: "The year I was 46 my periods just stopped without warning. They'd been as regular as clockwork until then, and I didn't have any hot flushes, irregularity or other signs that anything was changing. After six months without menstruating I had a period that was so heavy it was almost like a haemorrhage. I was flooding through tampons and towels so fast I couldn't go to work. The same thing happened again a month later, so I went to my G.P. who prescribed "Primolut" to control the bleeding. I took this for a couple of months, during which time I fell in love after being on my own for some years after my divorce. I went to the Family Planning clinic and asked to go back on the pill. This meant that I could not also take "Primolut" but the pill controlled the heavy bleeding as well as providing contraception. After five months I stopped taking the pill because my new relationship didn't work out. I never had another period and apart from the two very heavy periods I never had any symptoms or discomfort."

Joyce's experience was quite different: "I reached the age of 48 without really thinking about menopause. I was single, totally career-orientated and, if I thought about it at all, I thought a difficult menopause was something that happened to women who'd got nothing better to think about after their children left home. Well, I soon learnt otherwise! My periods began to get very heavy and pro-longed, sometimes lasting more than a week. Also my cycle got shorter, so the intervals between periods were shorter. When it reached the point where the periods were lasting ten days, with only two weeks "off" in between I went to my doctor who examined me, was pretty sure I had some big fibroids, and got me an appointment with a gynaecologist. She confirmed my own doctor's diagnosis, and suggested hysterectomy because the fibroids had got too big to remove otherwise. This took me by surprise a bit, but I was so exhausted from the almost continuous bleeding that I felt it would be the lesser of two evils. It took me longer than I expected to get over the surgery, but that was five years ago and I've been fine ever since."

Judith's experience was different again: "I have not menstruated now for well over a year, so I have to conclude that I am post-menopausal although I'm not yet 44. Three years ago my periods began to get very scanty. Whereas they had previously lasted 4 to 5 days with a fairly heavy flow on the first two days, they were over in three days. This went on for about 6 months getting lighter and lighter, although they were still quite regular, and then the intervals between each period began to get longer. Eventually they just dwindled away to nothing. I feel a bit sad, because it seems too soon for my fertile years to be over."

About a quarter of all women go through the menopause without any problems at all, and another quarter experience only minor difficulties which they feel able to handle alone. That leaves about 50% of women who feel the need for some help, from their doctor or other source and one aim of this book is to provide you with resources for finding such help, and also ways to help yourself.

The two most common problems of menopause for which women seek medical help are hot flushes (or flashes) and heavy bleeding.

As we have seen above, it is quite common for periods to get heavier for a while before they stop altogether. This may not amount to much more than a temporary nuisance but for some women the bleeding may verge on haemorrhage, making it difficult for them to carry on with everyday activities. If this goes on for any length of time, it is really debilitating and likely to make the woman very anaemic, so obviously professional help is needed.

Even such heavy bleeding, though, falls within the limits of "normal" and need not be a cause for worry. What is NOT normal is any bleeding between periods. During menopause, as at any age, such bleeding needs to be investigated promptly because it may be the first sign of illness that can be effectively treated if it is dealt with promptly. If periods are very irregular, how do you determine whether any loss of blood is "between" them? This is not as difficult as it may seem: if the bleeding is continuous, lasting at least a day to two days, it is almost certainly the next period, however long or short a time has passed since the last one but if there is just occasional "spotting" or bleeding which lasts for a few hours, stops and maybe starts again a few days later, it is not. You should also seek advice promptly if you experience bleeding after intercourse, or bleeding of any kind that happens a year or more after your last period.

Fibroids are a frequent cause of heavy bleeding, as you can see from Joyce's story. Fibroids are non-malignant lumps that form in or on the uterus. They have no connection with cancer. They are not a symptom of menopause, nor are they caused by it, but they often become a nuisance around this time. This is simply because they grow very slowly, and may take 20 years to reach a size where they cause discomfort or heavy bleeding, so a fibroid that has been form- ing since a woman was in her twenties will often come to light in her forties. Fibroid growth is influenced by oestrogen and small fibroids will often shrink and disappear without intervention at the end of menopause. There used to be a tendency among doctors to regard hysterectomy as the only treatment, however if the fibroids are small and not causing too much trouble, it is now considered a better policy to "wait and see". Small fibroids can also sometimes be removed surgically without removing the womb, but where they are large and deeply embedded in the tissue of the womb, hysterectomy may be the only practical solution. Although fibroids are quite often the cause of heavy bleeding, they do not cause bleeding between periods, so my earlier advice to have any such bleeding investigated holds good, even if you know that you have fibroids.

Hot flushes have become almost synonymous with menopause and are often regarded as a joke, though they are far from amusing to anybody who is experiencing them! The hot flush is, in fact, the single most common menopausal symptom, in spite of the fact that many women never have hot flushes at all.

Hot flushes are related to the amount of oestrogen circulating in the bloodstream. A sudden drop in oestrogen levels, such as happens when menopause is artificially induced (by removing the ovaries due to disease, for example) seems to trigger more severe flushing than a gradual decline.

The tiny blood vessels in the face, neck and sometimes the torso get bigger and extra blood rushes into them so that the woman feels very hot and her skin looks pink. This can last from a few seconds to several minutes and may happen as little as once or twice a week through to several times every hour. After the flushing, sweat usually breaks out, which cools the skin very quickly, creating a "yo-yo" effect of temperature rushing up and then down again.

The good news is that although hot flushes can be a real nuisance, and for some women a source of embarrassment, they are absolutely harmless! There is even a quite widely held belief that they are in some way "good for you" especially for the skin, but this seems to be a bit of an old wives' tale and I have not been able to find any evidence to support it. The only possible risk to health is when the flushes happen frequently during the night and stop the woman sleeping properly. If this goes on night after night it can obviously lead to extreme tiredness and some doctors have linked depression and mood-swings to this disturbance of sleep.

The problem usually tails off after a year or two, as the body adjusts to its new hormonal pattern, but in the most extreme cases it may continue for five or six years. Do remember, though, that these really are extreme cases and a great many women come to the end of menstruation without ever experiencing a hot flush.

The other physical changes which are attributable to lowered oestrogen levels take place far more slowly, and may not be experienced until quite a few years after menstruation has ended.

Loss of elasticity in the walls of the vagina, for example, is a very gradual process and so is the lessening of lubrication, so you may not notice any changes for a long time. The process can be slower still if you are able to maintain hormone levels to some extent (we'll be looking at how in the chapter on Hormones) and women who are sexually active experience these changes more slowly than those who are not. Contrary to the fear that many women have expressed to me, less lubrication does NOT mean a loss of desire, nor of the ability to reach orgasm. On the contrary, many menopausal and post-menopausal women find that they enjoy sex more than when they were younger.

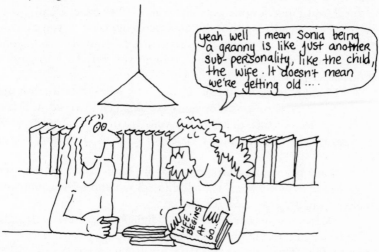

Prolapse of the womb affects some women in their fifties, sixties or later and is also something that develops slowly. It is as much linked to childbirth as to menopause and may have originated twenty or so years earlier. The uterus is partly supported by the pelvic floor muscles and partly by ligaments which cradle it rather like a sling and these ligaments and muscles may become stretched after giving birth, especially in women who have had several babies or a difficult delivery, though loss of muscle tone as we grow older contributes to the problem. Eventually the womb may drop down into the vagina, partly or wholly filling it. Alternatively, the womb may drop forwards, pressing on the bladder, or backwards, pressing on the rectum. In the worst cases the cervix may be visible outside the opening of the vagina, which leads to danger from infection as well as being very uncomfortable. If a prolapse is allowed to reach this extreme stage, surgery to reconstruct the internal support is usually the only practical solution but it is obviously better to do something about it long before that.

There is not much that can be done about stretched ligaments, but the pelvic floor muscles, fortunately, respond very well to exercise and strengthening them will prevent and even correct prolapse. You may be familiar with these exercises as part of a post-natal programme: if not, you can find details of how to do them in Part II of this book.

Loss of muscle-tone generally is also a slow process and lowering of oestrogen levels is not the only factor involved. If you exercise regularly you are obviously going to maintain good muscle tone longer than if you were sedentary, though you may have to work a little harder to do so.

Changes to skin and hair are only partly linked to lower levels of oestrogen. The processes of aging are as much involved, which is illustrated by the fact that women who have an abnormally early menopause do not become wrinkled or grey in their twenties or thirties.

Some of the other problems that are often associated with the menopause are not directly connected with the end of ovulation and the resulting drop in oestrogen.

Depression, anxiety and sexual difficulties are often thought of as being due to the physical changes, but there is no evidence to support this. These things are far more likely to result from other stresses in our lives that occur at roughly the same time. The only link between mental/emotional problems and what is happening in your body is that there is a tendency to be more emotionally reactive when hormone levels are fluctuating, such as in adolescence, during and shortly after pregnancy and (for some women) premenstrually. A study of women taking replacement hormones (in other words, ironing out the fluctuations) showed that this did not help those who were depressed.

All kinds of external circumstances can cause great stress during the mid-life years, for men as well as for women, so much so that the idea of "mid-life crisis" has become quite commonplace. For example, if you have spent most of your adult life bringing up children, the time when the last child leaves home can bring a feeling of emptiness and uselessness. A woman who has not had any children may experience grief when the time comes that she no longer has the physical ability to do so. Career women in their 40's to 50's often face very challenging situations: they may be competing with men, or with younger women, for promotion or, conversely, be facing the prospect of redundancy or compulsory early retirement, both of which imply major financial worries.

This is often the time in our lives when our parents, or other older relatives, die and apart from the inevitable grieving, this may raise issues around our own mortality. The birth of our first grandchildren can also bring up fears about aging and eventually dying, even as we delight in the new baby and share our children's pleasure.

These are factors that affect men just as much as women, even though men do not have a physical menopause. (They continue to produce sperm throughout their lives, and levels of the main male hormone, testosterone, vary very little. The phrase "male menopause" is strictly speaking, 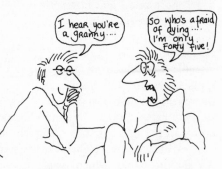 inaccurate.) It is only because these things often happen to coincide with the period of physical change for women that they have become linked with menopause in many people's minds.

There are many other problems that can arise as complications of menopause, but they are so rare that only a few women in many thousands are likely to experience any of them. I don't propose to discuss them here - this is not a medical encyclopaedia! Use this chapter as a guide to what you are likely to experience, and seek professional advice on anything that falls outside the norm.

3

A BIT ABOUT YOUR HORMONES

Our hormones take the blame for an awful lot! If our teenage off-spring are sulky and spotty, it's their hormones, if a pregnant or breastfeeding mother feels weepy, it's her hormones, and if a middle-aged woman is depressed or putting on weight, it's her hormones again. In fact, in each of these examples changing levels of hormones in the body **MIGHT** be involved, but which hormones? and how do they affect our skin, or our weight, let alone our emotions? It is equally possible that the teenage spots are due to junk food, the nursing mother's weeps to sheer exhaustion and the middle-aged woman's depression due to events in her life. The most frequent scenario is that bad diet, tired-ness or life changes coincide with a time when hormone levels are fluctuating wildly, which makes people more feel more vulnerable and reactive.

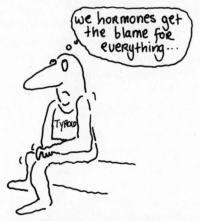

In order to understand the role of hormones in menopause, it is worth taking a little time to look at what hormones are and how they work in our bodies.

Hormones are often described as "chemical messengers" and the messages that they carry are the triggers that control many func-tions of the body. How fast you grow, how efficiently you convert the food you eat into energy, even how much urine you produce is influenced by hormones. The hormones of the reproductive system trigger the development of secondary sexual characteristics at puberty – the appearance of pubic and underarm hair, the growth of breasts and widening of the hips in girls and deepening voice and growth of facial hair in boys – as well as controlling the menstrual cycle.

These reproductive hormones are the ones mainly involved in the changes that take place during the menopause and after, but no single hormone acts in isolation: they interact with each other, sometimes in very complex ways, so it helps in understanding the menopausal changes if we know a bit about the system as a whole.

Hormones are produced in a number of glands which make up the Endocrine System (see Diagram 1) and released into the bloodstream as they are needed. They may affect the whole body or the working of a particular organ. The gland where the hormone originates may or may not be near the organ it affects as you will see from the following outline of the various gland, the hormones they produce and what these hormones do.

THE ENDOCRINE GLANDS AND WHAT THEY DO

The Pituitary Gland

The Pituitary gland, near the bottom of the brain, is the "master gland" which regulates the interaction of the other glands. It produces a lot of different hormones. Some of them act directly on the body and some of them work indirectly by triggering off the action of other endocrine glands.

Pituitrin directly regulates growth. Too much or too little leads to excessive height or stunted growth. If too much is produced once a person has reached adulthood it causes abnormal outgrowths of bone.

Thyroid stimulating hormone (TSH) controls the metabolism indirectly, by governing the Thyroid gland.

Adrenocorticotrophic hormone (ACTH) stimulates the part of the Adrenal glands that makes cortisone, hydrocortisone, etc.

Follicle stimulating hormone (FSH) regulates the production of sperm in men and ova (eggs) in women as well as the production and release of oestrogen from the ovaries.

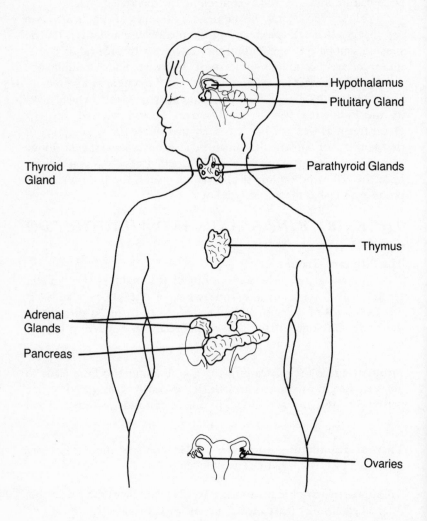

Diagram 1. The Endocrine Glands – Our Hormone Makers.

Luteinizing hormone (LH) regulates the ripening and release of ova, the production of progesterone in women and testosterone in men.

Oxytocin triggers the contractions of the uterus during labour.

Prolactin is involved in the production of breast milk.

Vasopressin works on the muscles of the bladder and intestines. It also constricts blood vessels (i.e. makes them smaller) leading to a temporary rise in blood pressure.

Antidiuretic hormone works on the kidneys and reduces the amount of water in the urine.

The Adrenal Glands

The Adrenals, just above the kidneys, also produce several different hormones:

Adrenalin is secreted from these glands when we are anxious or frightened. It prepares the body for vigorous activity (because when our distant ancestors were evolving, stressful situations usually called for physical action – fighting or running away fast). Nowadays the solution to a stressful situation seldom calls for physical action, so the adrenalin goes on circulating in our bloodstream for some time, often making us feel quite ill.

Cortisone and **Hydrocortisone** are produced in a different part of the Adrenals. These hormones help to turn starches in our food into simple sugars that our bodies can utilize. They are also involved in the ability of our skin to heal, especially in the case of allergies.

The Adrenals also make small amounts of **Oestrogen** (an important fact after the menopause when the ovaries no longer do so) and some other male and female hormones.

The Thyroid Gland

The Thyroid, at the base of the neck, makes **Thyroxin** which regulates our metabolism – the rate at which we "burn up" our food.

The Parathyroid Glands

The four Parathyroids, two on each side of the Thyroid, make **Parathormone** which regulates the amount of calcium in the bloodstream.

The Islets of Langerhans

These are found in the Pancreas, and they secrete **Insulin**. This regulates the level of sugar in the blood.

The Thymus Gland

The Thymus, in the upper chest secretes **Thymosin** which helps the immune system. This gland is a kind of bridge between the Endocrine system and the Lymphatic system (which helps our bodies fight infection, as well as draining fluids from the tissues).

The Ovaries and Testes

These produce the male and female hormones (as well as sperm and eggs). In fact, we all have some of each of these hormones. Men have small amounts of "female" hormones and women small amounts of "male" hormones.

Testosterone, the main male hormone triggers the development of sexual organs at puberty, as well as deepening of the voice, growth of body hair, beard, etc. It **governs the production of sperm and the amount of testosterone circulating in the blood** affects the sexual "drive" or libido. Testosterone also affects muscle tone, giving men some advantage over women in terms of muscular strength. The small amount of testosterone that women produce is also related to their sexual drive.

Oestrogen and **Progesterone** are responsible for the development of secondary female sexual characteristics – breast development, softer facial skin, absence of facial hair. **They operate in a delicate balance with FSH and LH to regulate the menstrual cycle.** Production of oestrogen and progesterone falls sharply at the menopause as ovulation (the production of eggs) declines. During the early stages of menopause, the Pituitary gland sends out more Follicle Stimulating Hormone to try and re-start the process of ovulation.

As you can see, the Endocrine system is very complex. It is kept in balance overall by a system of feedback. Although, as you have seen, the Pituitary gland is the master gland, the Pituitary itself is closely connected to a structure at the base of the brain, called the Hypothalamus which constantly monitors the effects of all the various hormones and influences the Pituitary as needed to keep them all working harmoniously. The Hypothalamus is sometimes called "the interface between mind and body" because it controls many of our body systems, but it is intimately linked to the part of our brain which seems to be mostly concerned with our emotions. So it comes about that our hormones can affect our emotions, and our emotions can affect our hormones.

This is a very simple outline of what our endocrine glands do, but it isn't the end of the story. What happens to the hormones in your bloodstream once they have done their work? Some of them are broken down in the liver and excreted, but the human body is a very efficient machine and avoids waste whenever possible, so a lot of re-cycling goes on. "Used" hormones are often converted into different hormones and other substances useful to the body, while conversely the glands sometimes use materials that would otherwise be wasted or even harmful, to manufacture hormones and this is why changing hormone levels can affect your body in so many different ways.

For example, cholesterol from the bloodstream is used in making oestrogens, so when the ovaries stop producing oestrogen, the cholesterol levels in the blood may rise, increasing the risk of heart disease. Oestrogen and other hormones are also involved in the process of fixing calcium in our bones. These facts are very important in understanding what happens to our bodies after the menopause, because heart disease and osteoporosis ("brittle bone disease") are two serious conditions linked to lowered oestrogen levels.

HORMONES AND THE MENOPAUSE

Some of the problems that women experience during menopause are directly due to the fact that the ovaries stop producing female hormones. Some other problems may be indirectly linked to lower levels of oestrogen and still others have no connection at all with hormones – they simply happen at the same time – but very often get blamed on "the change".

When the ovaries stop producing eggs, or ova, regularly, the amount of oestrogen they produce decreases considerably and this drop in the amount of oestrogen circulating in the body gives rise, directly or indirectly, to all the other changes in the body.

When oestrogen levels first begin to fall – especially if they do so rapidly, the Pituitary gland puts out more Follicle Stimulating Hormone (FSH) in an attempt to "kick-start" the ovaries into action. This leads to an excessive amount of FSH in the bloodstream at times, combined with too little oestrogen. (If a woman is not certain whether she is experiencing menopause, a blood-test which shows the relative levels of FSH and Ostrogen is a sure diagnosis.)

This imbalance between the various hormones can give rise to hot flushes, night sweats, irregular menstruation and heavy bleeding.

The degree to which they are experienced appears to be connected with the speed at which the oestrogen levels fall. Women who have had an "artificial menopause" when their ovaries were surgically removed or made inactive by chemotherapy because of disease often experience far more hot flushes than those whose periods end naturally, and this suggests that the suddenness of oestrogen reduction is involved.

Some longer-term consequences of menopause, such as vaginal dryness are due more simply to the lower amount of oestrogen in the body.

The body does not stop making oestrogen altogether once ovulation ends: the adrenal glands produce sex hormones throughout life, in both men and women. Another hormone manufactured by the adrenal glands is converted into oestrone (a form of oestrogen) in the fat cells. The more fat, the more constant the oestrogen levels will remain. As a result, plump women often experience an easier menopause than thin ones. But don't rush out and binge on cream buns – that will only increase the risk of a heart attack! The ovaries continue to make small amounts of testosterone after menopause, and this is quite important for a woman's wellbeing.

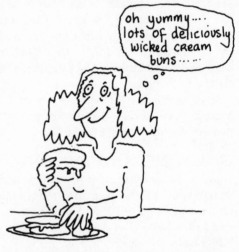

oh yummy.... lots of deliciously wicked cream buns....

So, to sum up, some of the discomforts and problems of menopause are directly due to lowered levels of oestrogen and progesterone in the body, some are indirectly connected to the reduction in these hormones, and some have nothing to do with hormone levels.

4

THE HEART OF THE MATTER

A S I HAVE said earlier, none of the discomforts or health problems
that some women experience during menopause are actually
damaging but there are two long-term results of lower oestrogen
levels in the body that do have serious implications. One of these is
osteoporosis and the other is the increased risk of heart disease.

Women in their reproductive years have only half as much risk
of heart disease as men in their age group, but after menopause this
risk gradually increases until the risks are the same for both men and
women. The reasons for this lie mainly in the effect of oestrogen on
the blood vessels.

One effect of oestrogen in the body is to increase the elasticity
of many kinds of body tissue and the reason nature "designed" us
this way is to facilitate pregnancy and childbirth. The elasticity of the
womb itself enables it to stretch to accommodate the growing foetus.
A pregnant woman's blood vessels need to expand to cope with
the increased amount of blood in her circulation – her own and the
foetus's. If her arteries and veins were as inelastic as a man's, high
blood pressure would kill her and her baby around the fifth month of
pregnancy. Whether you have had any pregnancies or not makes no
difference: the amount of eostrogen in your body throughout your
reproductive years is enough to keep your blood vessels elastic.

When we get to the end of our child-bearing years, we have
less oestrogen circulating round the body and our tissues, including
the blood vessels, gradually become less elastic. From the point of
view of having babies, this doesn't matter any more, but it does affect
other aspects of our health. As the walls of our blood vessels lose
some of their elasticity, we run a greater risk of high blood pressure
and heart disease.

The other factor involved is that our bodies – wonderful re-
cycling plants that they are – actually use cholesterol to manufacture

oestrogen. Less oestrogen being made means more cholesterol circulating in the body, so there is more risk of fatty deposits sticking to the walls of the arteries.

Hardening of the artery walls and narrowing of the arteries by fatty deposits are the two things that lead to heart attacks. All muscles need oxygen and nutrients to act as "fuel" to keep them working and these are carried to the muscles in the blood-stream. The heart is a powerful muscle which never stops working from well before our birth until the moment of death so it needs an unending supply of these fuels. Oxygenated blood is carried to the heart by the coronary arteries but if they become hardened or narrowed because their walls are coated with fatty deposits of cholesterol, less blood can pass through and the heart is literally "starved" of the oxygen it needs in order to function properly. Symptoms may include dizziness, difficulty in breathing and pain in the chest, which sometimes spreads to the arms, neck and midriff. This kind of pain, angina, usually goes away with rest but it serves a very important purpose in alerting the sufferer to the fact that something is wrong. Taking heed of such warning, and doing something about it, can avert a heart attack later.

A heart attack, or coronary thrombosis, happens when a blood clot gets stuck in a coronary artery that is already narrowed and blocks it completely. This cuts off all supply of blood to a section of the heart muscle which quite literally "suffocates" without its supply of oxygen. This usually causes intense pain and the heart may stop beating. Some people die within minutes, but contrary to the popular notion about heart attacks, these are the minority. Most people survive, though the next few days are a dangerous time and they need expert nursing during the next two to three weeks. Most people recover within about six weeks but there is then the danger that, if nothing is done to remedy the underlying condition, they will have another heart attack, and that one is more likely to be fatal.

When the health of the blood-vessels has deteriorated this badly, treatment may involve angioplasty, where a balloon is passed through the artery and inflated to widen the narrowed area. If the condition of the arteries is too poor to allow that, a coronary by-pass may be done. This involves taking a length of healthy vein from else-where in the body and grafting it into the coronary artery to by-pass the blocked section. But surgery does not change the conditions within the body that lead to the deterioration of the arteries in the first place, and unless major changes in lifestyle are made, a third of all coronary by-passes become blocked again within ten years, and the same proportion of arteries treated by angioplasty will have narrowed again in six months.

Both orthodox and alternative health professionals agree that prevention is by far the better course of action. This is true for both men and women and at any stage in life, but for menopausal and post-menopausal women it is doubly important, as they lose the protection from heart-disease which oestrogen provides.

You can see how much the heart depends on the state of the blood-vessels that supply it, and this aspect of our well-being is usually referred to as our cardiovascular health: "cardio" meaning "to do with the heart" and "vascular" "to do with the veins and arteries". Preventing heart disease is largely a question of keeping the veins and arteries in good condition and the two aspects of lifestyle which have the greatest impact are our old friends, diet and exercise. You'll find some detailed suggestions about both in Part II. If you have ex-perienced any warning signs or a cholesterol test has shown that you have dangerously high levels in your blood, don't expect lifestyle changes to produce results immediately. It may be several weeks or even months before you feel the benefit -but remember that it has taken many years for your health problem to develop and be patient. Even if you decide to take drugs to help, they will be more effective if you make some changes in your lifestyle as well.

Another major factor is smoking. Nicotine damages cardio-vascular health in several ways: it decreases the elasticity of the artery walls and reduces the amount of oxygen reaching the heart in the bloodstream. This is because carbon monoxide in cigarette smoke replaces some of the oxygen in the blood.

Maintaining a sensible weight is important, too, because excess weight places undue strain on the heart. This doesn't mean crash dieting (which is really bad for your health in the long term) or trying to look like an anorexic mannequin. If you avoid the foods that are damaging to your heart you will probably find it very easy to keep your weight at a healthy level.

As we have seen, your heart is a muscle and like all muscles it gets stronger the harder you make it work. Your heart does work continuously, of course, from long before you are born until you take your last breath but it needs harder work than that to keep it healthy. Human bodies evolved to meet the physical demands made on early humans: walking long distances, hunting, running, lifting and carrying heavy loads. Our "easy" 20th century lifestyle seldom gives the body enough to do and our hearts suffer as a result, unless we build in some exercise to compensate.

Exercise helps your heart in several ways: it increases the flow of blood to the heart, and therefore the amount of oxygen it gets from your lungs, it makes your heart "work" a little harder and if you have excess pounds (which put an extra strain on the heart) it will help you to lose them. In addition, we now know that regular exercise even alters the composition of fats in your bloodstream. Regular exercisers have less of the damaging cholesterol and more of the "good" fats that carry cholesterol to the liver, where it is broken down for excretion.

I realise that many of these suggestions can sound very negative and suspiciously like nagging. Perhaps the most positive thing I can say is that you have the ability to add several decades to your lifespan, and healthy decades, at that. Heart disease is a major cause of premature death, and you CAN do something about it.

THE FEELING HEART

So far, I have only talked about the physical factors that influence the health of the heart but we need to consider mental and emotional factors, too.

The idea that stress, anxiety and shock contribute to heart disease is no fallacy. When we experience mental or emotional stress our adrenal glands respond by producing adrenalin and other hormones which increase the activity of the heart muscle and temporarily raise blood pressure. This prepares the body for strenuous physical action and our bodies respond in such a way because when we were evolving a stressful situation was usually one that demanded physical action. If we don't react with a physical activity, such as fighting or running away, we are left with a thumping heart and adrenalin circulating in the body uselessly, which places strain on the heart, adrenal glands and other organs. If this happens occasionally, the body can usually readjust quite quickly, but repeated or continuous stress is really damaging, for example, high blood pressure can become an ongoing problem which increases the risk of heart disease.

The stresses in contemporary life are seldom solved by a physical response so, to safeguard our health, we need to find other strategies for dealing with stressful situations.

Some people reduce the harmful effects of stress by taking

vigourous exercise. Smashing a squash ball about burns up the adrenalin just as effectively as smashing in your rival's skull!

Alternatively, we can look at ways of reducing the impact of stress on the body through activities that counteract stress, such as meditation, specific relaxation techniques or yoga (and almost every yoga class will include a period of relaxation and/or meditation). There are many different kinds of meditation and you may need to try several before you discover the form that you feel most at home with. There are plenty of books and tapes available but it is probably easier to learn from an experienced meditator. This might be somebody who is formally teaching meditation, or simply a friend who has been practising for a while.

If you can't find anybody to teach you, you may like to try the following simple meditation on the breath:

Sit comfortably with your back upright. It doesn't matter whether you sit in a chair or on the floor so long as your spine is straight. Take a few minutes to settle down and then begin to notice your breath. Don't do anything to change it, like breathing more deeply or slowly: just notice it.

Now start counting your breaths. Breathe in, breathe out and count "one", breathe in, breathe out, count "two" and so on, up to ten. When you get to ten, go back to one and start again. If you lose track of the numbers, start again at one. Try not to think about anything else except breathing. If you find yourself thinking about anything else, just go back to one and start counting your breaths again. All sorts of thought will creep in, of course, but don't feel that you are failing with the meditation when that happens. Just recognise that some thought has arisen but don't follow it through. For example: you hear a door banging, simply register "I heard a door banging", don't get involved with "Which door was it? Why was it banging? Did somebody slam it? Who was it?". This may feel hard at first, but the more often you practise the easier it gets to put thoughts aside.

This is only one form of meditation on the breath: there are many others, and all are equally valid. This is an easy one to start with because the counting gives you something to concentrate on. When you have practised this for some time, you can try leaving out the counting. Just focus on your breathing, notice the breathe as it enters your nose, notice how your chest and belly move when you breathe in and when you breathe out, notice the breathe as it leaves your nose.

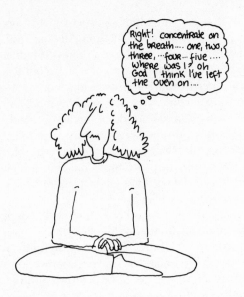

Many physical tests have been carried out which show that during meditation the heartbeat slows down, high blood pressure is lowered and brain rhythms become very stable. Even if these effects only last for the length of the meditation they are beneficial, but in fact they persist for some time after, and the more regularly a person meditates the longer the physical effects last. Try to meditate every day, starting with perhaps five to ten minutes each day, and increase that to twenty minutes if possible.

Although meditation is such an effective way to counteract stress, a time when you are under a lot of stress is not the best time to start learning to meditate. It helps if you can master a technique during a relatively calm period. Don't think of meditation as something you can take like a dose of aspirin when the going gets rough! Try, rather, to meditate for the sake of meditating without looking for "results" otherwise it can become just another source of stress.

Be kind to your feeling heart. If you are emotionally distressed, don't bottle it up. Cry, rage, find a trusted friend you can talk to. If your distress is greater than can be helped in such simple ways, you might think about asking counselling or some form of psychotherapy. Remember that you don't have to be mentally ill to benefit from such help and there is no stigma attached to asking for help if you need it. Be gentle. Try to cultivate an open and loving attitude to other people as much as you can. Yes, I know it isn't always easy.

Finally, enjoy yourself! Give yourself permission to have fun.

Your heart will thank you.

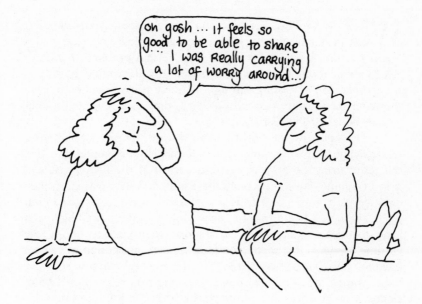

5

I FEEL IT IN MY BONES

WHEN WAS THE last time you thought about your bones? It was probably quite a long time ago, unless you have had a recent fracture, joint pain or other bone-related problem. We don't usually think about our bones unless they give us trouble, but if you are approaching or passing through the menopause – and even more so if your menopause is completed – it is time to give some thought to your bones BEFORE they give you trouble.

Osteoporosis, or "brittle-bone disease" is one of the most severe,debilitating and potentially life-threatening conditions that can result from the drop in oestrogen levels at the menopause and it is becoming far more common (about one-third of all women now develop osteoporosis, four times as many as a generation ago). The bones begin to lose calcium and become more fragile and likely to fracture more easily. As the disease progresses, bones may become so vulnerable that a cough or a sneeze is enough to cause a fracture. This can be considered "life-threatening" because so many older women die of complications following major fractures. 12% of elderly women who suffer hip fractures die in the following months. Perhaps more important, though, is the diminished quality of life osteoporosis can cause, due to fragility, loss of mobility and often of independence.

It is sometimes called "the invisible epidemic" because there is nothing to show that the bones are getting more fragile. The first sign is often a fractured wrist when a woman trips and puts out an arm to save herself. This will usually heal in 6 to 8 weeks, but should be seen as an alarm signal, and everything possible done to prevent further bone loss before more serious fractures follow. The most common fractures, apart from the wrist, are of the spinal vertebrae and the hip (or neck of the femur). The femur is the long, strong bone forming your thigh, but at the point where it fits into the socket of your hip, it is much narrower. This narrow section carries a great deal of your body weight, so it is particularly vulnerable.

A very disabling form of osteoporosis involves crumbling of the spine. When a lot of calcium is lost from the vertebrae they collapse, shortening the spine and making it bend forwards. Can you picture a "little old lady", bent double over her walking stick and no taller than an average ten-year old? She may have been an upright and stately 5"7' before osteoporosis destroyed her spine. What you can't immediately see is that her lungs are compressed, making breathing difficult, her stomach and other digestive organs are compressed, too, because as the spine bends forwards the lower ribs are pushed down, sometimes so far that they rest on the hip bones. She may even have had her lower ribs surgically removed to reduce the pressure on her pelvis. Not surprisingly, this old lady is in more or less constant pain.

BUT IT DOESN'T HAVE TO BE LIKE THAT. The good news is that OSTEOPOROSIS IS, TO A LARGE DEGREE, PRE-VENTABLE and most of the preventive measures are THINGS YOU CAN DO FOR YOURSELF.

You'll see that I have said it is **"to a large degree"** preventable because everybody's bones thin to some extent as they get older, men's as well as women's. What **can** be prevented in most cases is the dramatic thinning that leads to abnormal fractures.

You don't often see men suffering from severe osteoporosis, though cases do occur. There are several reasons for this: men's bones are generally larger than women's to start with and the amount of oestrogen circulating in their bloodstream is more or less constant throughout life. Oestrogen is involved in the body processes that help to fix calcium in the bones so the big drop in oestrogen levels at menopause is a major factor leading to bone loss in women. A third factor is that women in general live longer than men, so there is simply more time for the effects of calcium loss to show up.

We all, men and women alike, build bone during the earlier part of our lives – who hasn't been told in childhood to drink up their milk because it makes strong bones? This bone-building peaks somewhere around 35 when the bones have reached their maximum size and density. This is known as the peak bone mass. After 35 the bones start to thin, though it will be many years before there is any outward sign of this. Even on X-ray it is difficult to see any difference until about one-third of bone mass has been lost. More sophisticated methods of measuring bone-loss have been devised, but they are available in only a few centres.

The best way to treat osteoporosis is to prevent it, and the earlier you embark on a programme of preventive measures, the more effective they will be. Ideally, women should start protecting their bones before they reach their peak mass in the mid-thirties so if you have daughters or granddaughters, pass on all this information to them – the teens are not too soon to start taking care of your bones. But if you are experiencing your menopause now or if it is completed, you can still do a lot to strengthen your bones so let's start NOW by thinking a bit about our bones and how they work. Understanding that will make sense of the how and why of keeping them healthy.

WHAT BONES ARE MADE OF

Most of us, if we think about bones at all, tend to think of them as inert, solid masses. The image that most likely springs to mind is the desiccated skeleton that hung in the biology lab at school, or something the dog dug up, but those of course are long-dead bones. The bones that support you as you read this as are just as alive as any other part of your body and, like all living tissue, they are constantly changing. Bone tissue dies and is replaced with new tissue all the time, just like the rest of your body.

Bones have a tough outer layer and a more porous inner layer, rather like a honeycomb. (If they were solid all the way through, they would be so heavy we could hardly move!) They are made up of a number of minerals: calcium, phosphorus, magnesium and smaller amounts of others. Calcium, which forms the largest part is the commonest mineral on Earth, taking many forms from the scale that forms in your kettle to exquisite crystals, via stalactites, stalagmites and towering chalk cliffs. In fact, our bones are the part of ourselves which most resemble our mother Earth, or Gaia. Bones are not only made of the same minerals as crystals, they are themselves crystalline structures – the calcium that forms much of your bones is actually in the form of myriads of microscopic crystals.

We cannot make any of these minerals within our bodies, so we have to get them from our food. Munching a bit of rock is not an efficient way of absorbing calcium, so we depend on the plant kingdom to help us. Plants absorb calcium and other minerals from the Earth and convert them into forms our bodies can use. (And the reason why milk is such a good source of calcium is that cows eat an awful lot of grass!)

Once we have digested the calcium and other minerals, they are carried to the different parts of our body in the bloodstream. Bones have their own blood supply from which they absorb the nutrients they need, but sometimes nutrients can be taken out of the bones if they are more urgently needed in some other part of the body. Most of the time, 99% of the calcium in our bodies is held in the bones while the other 1% circulates in the blood ready to supply other organs. Our brains cannot function without calcium, and we also need some in our muscles. So if the amount in the bloodstream falls much below 1% our ever-wise bodies "steal" calcium from the bones to prevent the brain going short.

The minerals that make up our bones are "glued" together by collagen. Collagen is fairly elastic and gives the bones some flexibility, which makes them less liable to break. But collagen gets less elastic as we grow older. It is an important part of your skin, too, and saggy, wrinkled skin is another result of collagen losing its elasticity. Collagen needs Vitamin C to keep it healthy and elastic, so another bone-protecting measure is getting enough of this vitamin, and it will help to keep your skin in good condition, too.

HOW TO PROTECT YOUR BONES

One of the first steps towards protecting your bones is making sure you get enough calcium and other minerals from your food and the vitamins that help your body use that calcium effectively.

As you have already seen, oestrogen plays a part in the chemical processes that fix calcium in the bones. Less oestrogen means less fixing of calcium, so another bone-protecting strategy is doing whatever you can to maintain oestrogen levels after the ovaries stop making it.

The third thing you can do to protect your bones is to make them work harder! We are all used to the idea that exercise makes your muscles stronger: the evidence is there to be seen. We are less used to the notion that exercise can strengthen the bones and of course we can't see what is happening to them.

The bones that make up your skeleton have two main functions: to protect vital organs and to provide a framework around which your muscles can work. Almost every muscle in your body is attached to bones at two or more points and every time the muscles move, they pull on the bones. The bones respond to this by increasing their bulk to withstand the pull from the muscles. So, the more you use your muscles, the stronger your bones become – simple, isn't it?

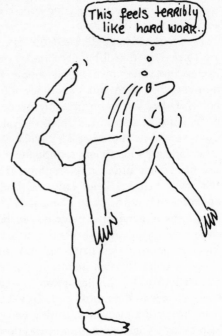

Our bodies were designed for plenty of physical activity, and some doctors believe that the alarming increase in osteoporosis is due to the fact that modern life is less physically demanding than it was in earlier times.

Plenty of exercise **before** that crucial slowing-down point in the mid-thirties is a big factor in preventing bone disease later, but even if you are already well past that point, regular exercise is one of the most important things you can do to maintain the health of your bones. In fact, many authorities think exercise is the single most important factor influencing bone strength. Studies of women **already suffering with osteoporosis** have shown how much they can strengthen their bones through suitable exercise. Obviously, if the bones are already weak, this must be done on medical advice and under proper supervision.

To sum up so far, the strength of your bones depends on:

The amount of calcium and other minerals and vitamins you get from your food.

The amount of exercise you take.

The amount of oestrogen in your body.

The first two factors are **entirely within your own control.** You, and only you, can determine what you eat and what exercise you take. Oestrogen levels aren't quite so easily controlled, but even so there are sensible steps you can take to maintain them. Most of these have been described elsewhere in this book, in the chapter on hormones or under the heading of the various therapies that can help, so I will not go into them again in detail.

Being in a high-risk category for osteoporosis is one of the most frequent reasons for using HRT and for some women it may be a sensible choice as it does prevent bone-loss by keeping oestrogen levels steady for as long as the replacement hormones are taken. The levels will drop immediately HRT is discontinued and some doctors think that the therapy should be continued indefinitely. Others feel that it can safely be discontinued after some 10 or 12 years, if started in the mid-40's, because it will have delayed bone-loss long enough for no ill effects to be apparent during the woman's likely lifetime.

Many women dislike the idea of indefinite drug-taking, and if you are not in a high-risk category (which I shall go into a little later) good nutrition, regular exercise and non-drug ways of maintaining oestrogen are safer. Even if you do opt for HRT good nutrition and some form of exercise are important and may make it possible for you to take lower doses of the drugs because the three factors we have been looking at all interact. As I mentioned in Chapter 11, there are some women who cannot be given HRT at all because of other health problems and for them non-drug methods of maintaining bone mass are essential.

ARE YOU AT RISK?

It helps to know whether you fall into a high-risk category or not, as this may be crucial in deciding whether or not the risks involved in taking HRT are outweighed by the risk of abnormal fractures and their complications.

If you are a petite, small boned woman you are at greater risk than a larger woman with a heavy frame because your peak bone mass is less, so calcium loss can thin your bones to a dangerous extent much sooner. The heavier woman is also "loading" her bones more effectively, simply because of the additional weight they carry.

If you take little exercise, and particularly if you took very little exercise before you reached your mid-30's your risk is greater, as exercise increases bone mass. So the petite woman in our first example may actually have stronger bones than her heavier neighbour, if she took – and still takes – plenty of bone-loading exercise.

A very early menopause increases risk, because the earlier your oestrogen levels begin to fall the earlier your bones start to lose calcium.

Total hysterectomy (including removal of the ovaries) or surgical removal of the ovaries alone due to disease, brings about an artificial menopause as oestrogen production from the ovaries stops abruptly. This, too, increases the risk of osteoporosis, especially if surgery takes place before the average age of menopause. The drop in oestrogen levels is sudden, and loss of bone-mass can take place much faster than when hormone levels fall gradually. The same is true when the ovaries have been rendered inactive by radiation or chemotherapy.

There is a hereditary or genetic factor: if your mother, grandmother or other older women relatives suffered abnormal fractures you may be at greater risk. Don't get too hung up on this one, though: the crippled great-aunt may have eaten a calcium-deficient diet and led a very sedentary life. You know better and can avoid those mistakes, though we often "inherit" bad eating habits and lifestyles as much as our family's genes. Look around the family and see whether there are **a number** of older women with brittle bones: if so, you would be wise to consider the genetic factor.

A genetic factor which cannot be confused with lifestyle or diet is your ethnic origin. European women, particularly if they are blonde and fair skinned, are at greater risk than African and Mediterranean women. Asian women fall somewhere in between. The highest incidence of osteoporosis is found in the UK, Switzerland and Scandinavia where people consume a lot of dairy products and this suggests that factors other than calcium intake are involved.

Women who have not had any babies are at more risk than those who have, though teenage pregnancies increase risk because calcium is diverted to the foetus before the mother has finished growing herself.

There are also some aspects of lifestyle that increase risk.

Poor diet and lack of exercise are two of these, as you've already seen. Heavy use of alcohol, coffee, cigarettes, cola drinks and junk food are some others.

If you have suffered from anorexia, or have dieted drastically to lose weight, especially if you've done so often, also increases risk. Women athletes, runners and dancers who train excessively and stop menstruating are at increased risk, because their oestrogen productions stops, too.

YOUR CHANCES OF DEVELOPING BRITTLE BONES ARE GREATER IF:

You are a fair-skinned woman of European origin.

You are slim and small boned.

You have had no children or you have had a baby in your teens.

You had an early menopause.

You have had your ovaries removed surgically, especially if this was before the average age of menopause.

Other women in your family had osteoporosis.

Your lifestyle is fairly sedentary.

Your diet is low in calcium.

You are or have been anorexic.

You have often crash-dieted to lose weight.

You have exercised so hard that your periods stopped.

You smoke, drink much coffee, alcohol or cola drinks or eat junk food.

YOUR CHANCES OF DEVELOPING BRITTLE BONES ARE LESS IF:

You are a dark-skinned woman of African or Mediterranean origin.

You are large and big-boned.

You have had one or more children.

Your menopause occurred later.

You take plenty of exercise.

Your diet is rich in calcium.

You avoid heavy use of alcohol, coffee, cigarettes and junk foods.

If any of the factors in the first list apply to you, don't panic, but do everything you can to protect your bones, and as quickly as possible. If you find that several factors in that list describe you or your lifestyle, do get professional advice. Whether you choose an orthodox medical approach, alternative therapies or a combination of both is a very personal matter, but whatever your decision, I beg you to use all the self-help methods outlined in this chapter as well.

If the second list seems more applicable to you – don't be too complacent! Keep up your exercise and your good diet, add some supplements if necessary and avoid the "baddies", if only because they affect many other aspects of your health, too.

FURTHER READING:

Bone Loading	Simkin & Alayon	*Prion*
Osteoporosis	Kathleen Mayes	*Thorsons*

6

THE UNKINDEST CUT

A COMPLAINT THAT I have often heard voiced about the medical profession is that doctors are far too ready to recommend hysterectomies, particularly for menopausal and post-menopausal women, when there may be other, less traumatic, ways of dealing with their health problems. Not all doctors are sensitive to the emotional and psychological implications of removing a woman's womb and take the attitude "It's not serving any useful purpose (i.e., having babies) any more, so you might as well get rid of it". This totally ignores the fact that, for many women, their womb is symbolic of their femaleness and to remove it is to take away a funda-mental part of their womanhood.

Even if we ignore the psychological aspect, hysterectomy is major surgery and recovery often takes longer than the six weeks quoted by surgeons.

Fortunately, this tendency has lessened since the introduction of hormone replacement therapy which is now seen as a panacea for many of the problems that were formerly thought of as reasons for removing the womb. This can only be good news since, whatever the arguments against HRT, it is at least reversible.

All the same, there are still doctors who are too quick to resort to the knife, so it is wise to know what other options are possible, and to ask for a second opinion and time to think if you are recom-mended surgery of this kind. If you want to try one of the natural therapies, such as homoeopathy or medical herbalism, for example, it may take several months before the benefits are noticeable so you might want to negotiate with your doctor along the lines of "If you can see a real improvement in my condition in 3 months time, will you reconsider your recommendation?" In any case, waiting time for surgery within the National Health Service is often so long that you could have plenty of time to see the results of alternative therapies, dietary changes, etc. before the date for your operation. You don't have to tell your doctor what you are doing if you think that prejudice about alternative therapies would affect his (or less often, her) attitude towards you and your treatment. But do ask to be re-examined if you feel that your condition has improved. If your doctor or gynaecologist agrees that there is improvement, that might be a good point at which to mention any other therapy you have been receiving. Who knows, you might even help to change a surgeon's mind about alternative therapies!

Fibroids are one of the conditions for which hysterectomy is often recommended. Fibroids often manifest at mid-life, not because they are in any way connected with the process of menopause but because they take many years to grow, and may only get large enough to be troublesome around this time. Doctors will often recommend a hysterectomy if fibroids are so big that they cause pain, pressure on other organs or abnormally heavy periods. If the fibroids are very large, and are deeply embedded in the walls of the uterus, hysterectomy may indeed be the right solution but if they are not deeply embedded, myectomy may be possible. This involves removing the fibroids while keeping the uterus intact but sometimes this form of operation proves to be so technically difficult that the surgeon may have to remove the whole womb, after all. Your gynaecologist should discuss this possibility with you beforehand.

If the fibroids are not causing great pain, or exerting a lot of pressure on other organs, it may be worth persevering with non-surgical methods of treatment because fibroids tend to shrink after menopause and you may well be able to avoid surgery altogether. If you experience heavy bleeding, your doctor should check your blood count regularly, to ensure against anaemia. You may need to take an iron supplement, but it is better to look for foods that provide you with plenty of iron, or if that is not sufficient, use a herbal iron supplement, as these are absorbed more easily by the body.

Herbal treatments have proved very successful in reducing fibroids, especially when combined with hydrotherapy and special exercises to improve circulation in the pelvic region. At a women's health centre in Geneva, every woman between 40 and 50 with fibroids showed improvement within six months when treated in this way, although some needed to continue the treatment for longer before they were completely free of symptoms. (I.e., the fibroids shrank until they no longer caused any problems.)

Hysterectomy may also be recommended for abnormally heavy menstrual bleeding due to causes other than fibroids. You might regard this approach as the sledgehammer to crack a nut, since there are many non-surgical treatments available, ranging from drug or hormone therapy through to herbal medicine, both Western and Oriental, that surgery should be viewed as the last resort if other methods prove ineffective. In such cases, there are less destructive forms of surgery available. One is the surgical laser which destroys the lining of the womb while leaving the womb itself intact. This is the most minimal form of surgery, and recovery usually takes only a few days. An alternative is cutting away the lining alone, with an instrument called a retroscope: this method, too, preserves the rest of the womb. However, you may not be offered these options as the techniques are relatively new and not all surgeons are familiar with them. If you really want to retain your womb, ask about these methods and whether you can be referred to a surgeon who uses them.

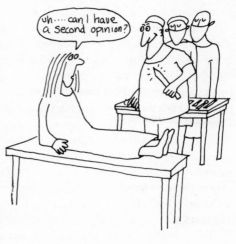

Not all women feel strongly about keeping their womb. Several years of pain, heavy bleeding or other complications may make the option of a hysterectomy seem like a welcome relief and it is true that some women do feel dramatically better after surgery. Conversely, some feel drained of energy and find recovery long and difficult and others feel that their femininity and sexuality have been diminished. It's important to discuss all these aspects beforehand. If you don't find it possible to discuss all the implications with your doctor or gynaecologist, it is worth seeking out somebody who can counsel you, perhaps at a well-woman clinic, a women's group or a natural health centre. Counselling can also be very helpful after a hysterectomy if you feel distressed in any way.

In some situations, such as uterine cancer, hysterectomy really is the best or only option but it is important to remember than many uterine cancers originate in the cervix (the neck of the womb) and only slowly invade the uterus itself. Abnormal changes (hyperplasia) in the cervical cells can be identified long before the cells become cancerous, and at that stage can be treated simply and successfully, both by orthodox and alternative methods. The system of cervical smear testing has been criticised, and it does have faults, but so far it is the best way we have of detecting hyperplasia before it develops into cancer so don't skip your three-yearly tests.

If you have been advised that a hysterectomy really is necessary, it is very important indeed to discuss with your doctor the question of leaving your ovaries. Some surgeons will remove the ovaries routinely when doing a hysterectomy "just in case" although if the ovaries are healthy at the time of the operation there is little risk of them becoming dis-eased later. A hysterectomy in which the ovaries are removed as well as the womb is referred to as a total hysterectomy so be alert to this when discussing a possible operation.

Keeping your ovaries if at all possible is really important for your long-term health and well-being. In fact, in terms of woman-hood and sexuality they are more important physically than the womb (although for some women the womb is more important psychologically and symbolically). Although the ovaries make very little oestrogen or progesterone once they stop producing eggs, they continue to secrete other hormones, called androgens, for a very long time, maybe until you are in your eighties. These hormones help to maintain muscular strength and elasticity, sex-drive and vaginal lubrication, so there are good reasons for hanging on to your ovaries unless there is a really valid reason for removing them. Some of the androgens are converted in the body into oestrogens, and as you already know maintaining oestrogen levels reduces the risk of osteoporosis as well as lessening problems such as hot flushes.

It may be genuinely necessary to remove the ovaries in cases of ovarian cancer, or if a benign ovarian cyst is very large and cannot be removed without damaging the ovary. Even so, it may be possible to leave the other ovary intact.

The younger you are at the time of any proposed surgery, the more important it is to preserve your ovaries if at all possible as the earlier the oestrogen levels are reduced, the greater the risk of osteoporosis later. Doctors may argue that this is easily remedied by replacement hormones but unless you are happy about the prospect of taking artificial hormones for the rest of your life, ask for a second opinion.

To sum up, hysterectomy is a major step and it is wise to consider all the advantages and disadvantages as well as all possible alternatives, surgical, drug or hormone based as well as the various forms of natural medicine, before making any decision. Your doctor owes it to you to discuss every aspect of the operation with you beforehand so that you can be well prepared both physically and psychologically. Women who have tried one of the natural therapies before deciding that surgery was the best option for them, often recover much faster but even if you opt for surgery without trying any alternatives, you can do a lot in terms of good diet, etc. to make sure your general health is good before any operation. This will almost certainly shorten your recovery time and reduce the risk of complications and you can still use good diet, appropriate exercise and all the options discussed in this book to maintain your health and vitality for many years to come.

Sandra's experience illustrates many of these points. She had a hysterectomy at the age of 40 because of extremely severe endometriosis. Part of her womb lining had ruptured and formed a sac within the uterus, so that she was bleeding from almost twice the normal inner surface of the womb. "I was bleeding for two weeks at a time, and for at least two days of that I couldn't go out." Sandra tried a number of different alternative therapies: healing, aromatherapy, homoeopathy all of which helped, but it was reflexology that helped most to reduce both the bleeding and the pain. "It also gave me the comforting touch of a hands-on therapy, but far enough away from the area to feel safe. All these therapies helped to keep me going, but they weren't enough to reverse the process. I certainly felt I was in better condition to have the operation as a result, and I was also wonderfully supported while I was in hospital as somebody came in to give me healing every day."

Sandra had a 9-month wait for her operation, which she felt gave her valuable time to get herself ready, both physically and emotionally: "The healing was part of letting go – being able to release my womb if I chose to. I came to understand that it was an essential part of me if I wanted to have children but not if I didn't, and I had no doubt at all that I did not want any more children. I didn't feel that it would diminish me as a woman. So I got to the point where I could say 'I have a choice, and I am choosing to do this.' As my consultant put it, my condition was not life-threatening but life-interruptive, and I wasn't prepared to plan my life around my menstrual cycle any more. You need to make your own decision, not be told what to do."

After the operation, Sandra went through some dramatic mood-swings, mainly because she found it very difficult to ask people to do things for her, to lie down and do nothing, when she'd always been the one to be doing things for other people. "It was a big lesson for me in being able to receive. Apart from that there weren't any emotional problems. I think I'd worked through it all before-hand. Physically, it took me about 6 months to feel fully recovered, though after 3 months I knew it had been a good thing for me. I didn't feel in any way less feminine because of it. I was a bit worried by some things I'd read in books about hysterectomy affecting your sex life but I was able to resume a normal love-life after the usual six weeks. In fact, after about 5 weeks it was a struggle not to make love!"

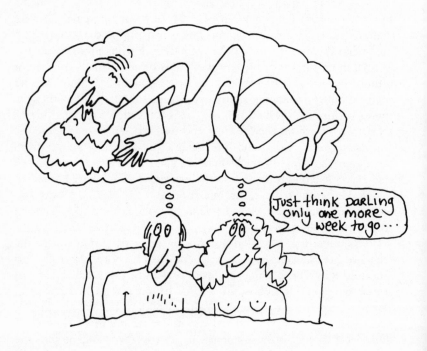

Some women do find a that hysterectomy affects their enjoyment of sex, especially if pressure on their womb during penetration was an important part of their pleasure before the operation, but almost of all of them rediscover their ability to enjoy sex and have orgasms. On the other hand, constant pain and/or abnormal bleeding are such a block to sexual pleasure that a hysterectomy can be the key to a whole new love life. In Sandra's words: "It was a relief to be freed from 'Not tonight darling, I'm bleeding.' It certainly released a lot of time and energy."

Finally, if you do have to have a hysterectomy, it isn't the end of the world. However important your womb is to you physically, or as a symbol of your womanhood, it is not YOU. Your essential, female, creative and loving self is not located in your physical body, but is part of that greater self for which your body is the vehicle.

FURTHER READING:

Natural Healing in Gynaecology	Rina Nissim	*Pandora*

7

SEX, LOVE AND RELATIONSHIPS

IN THE AUTUMN of 1989 I was in Los Angeles on my first visit to America, and my hosts took me to the preview of a new play, called "The Eighties". As we were nearing the end of the decade, we all assumed that would be the subject of the play but it was, in fact, about a couple in their eighties: he terminally ill, she losing her memory a bit. Towards the end of the second act, the old man proposed to his wife that they go to bed after lunch and make love. A round of nervous giggles ran round the audience. "But darling, you know you can't......" said the old lady. "I know what I can't do. I didn't say, let's go to bed and screw: I meant let's lie down together and pleasure each other". The laughter grew louder, and by the time the old man had suggested saving some of the soured cream from lunch "to put on each other so we can lick it off" the auditorium was in hysterics but the laughter had a brittle edge to it. Old people were not supposed to behave like this, not supposed to have sexual feeling and **certainly** not supposed to do anything that might be construed as "kinky". The gales of laughter hid a lot of un-comfortable feelings.

This little scene tells us a lot about the way society views the sexuality of older people: if the characters had been 50 years younger the conversation would have barely raised a titter.

The idea that older people – and particularly older women – don't enjoy sex is so deeply engrained in our minds that it colours women's expectations and it is clear from talking to a large number of women that the greatest area of anxiety about menopause is around this topic. Many fear that they will no longer enjoy sex once they stop menstruating, while others are afraid that they will no longer be attractive to their partners. Women who are married or in a long term relationship often express fear that their partner will lose interest in them and leave them for a younger woman. Those who are on their own through divorce, widowhood or other reasons fear being unable to attract a new partner.

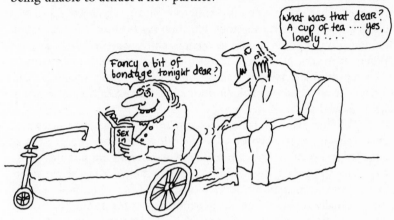

Most of these fears arise from social conditioning and they bear very little relationship to the known facts. Contrary to their earlier fears, many women enjoy sex more after the menopause and some who have not been able to reach orgasm before find that they can. The women I have talked to, almost without exception, attributed this delightful state of affairs to not having to worry about contraception (but do, please, see below). This is certainly a bonus for most women, but there may be other, less obvious, factors at play.

For example, quite a lot of women said that they felt inhibited about lovemaking when their children were growing up. By the time the children were old enough to stop creeping into their parents' bed for cuddles at all hours, they were also old enough to understand about sex, and some women felt shy or fearful of the children overhearing their lovemaking. This was particularly marked in the case of older teenagers and where offspring were still living at home into their early twenties. (It doesn't seem to operate in reverse, though, as one mother of several lusty sons remarked!) For these women, the departure of the last child from home had been sexually liberating: several said they felt able to initiate sex which they had not done before, or to make love in the daytime or in places other than their bedroom.

It is really important to understand that the physical and hormonal changes of the menopause have virtually no impact on a woman's ability to become sexually aroused and to reach orgasm.

The reproductive hormones, oestrogen and progesterone, which decrease in quantity at this time, have little influence on how sexy you feel. That is the role of testosterone and levels of this hormone do not vary much throughout life, but no hormone has as much influence on sexual response as mental, emotional and social factors. When an American research team studied a group of healthy women who reported a persistent lack of interest in sex, they found no difference at all between their hormones and those of a similar group who enjoyed sex.

Women who are taking replacement hormones (oestrogen and progesterone) often report that their love-life has improved, but when a group of women on HRT were carefully monitored, those who had reported a loss of interest in sex before they began treatment showed no improvement. Women on HRT may think it helps them sexually because they feel generally better for having their other problems alleviated. After all, nobody feels very amorous when they are disturbed by hot flushes and copious sweating night after night. (And that applies equally to a partner sharing the same bed!) Relieving the hot flushes by means other than HRT (aromatherapy, herbal medicine or homoeopathy, for example) is just as effective in restoring desire.

The physical changes that result from less oestrogen in the body have little effect on women's enjoyment of sex apart from the problem of vaginal dryness and this is very easily dealt with.

The decrease in lubrication does not, in itself, stop a woman wanting sex but what often happens is that making love becomes uncomfortable or difficult so she is fearful of trying again. Her partner may also avoid sexual contact because he is worried about the possibility of hurting her or he may initiate sex and then have difficultly getting an erection because of this worry. You see how easily misunderstandings can arise if partners don't talk to each other about what is happening: he thinks she has lost interest in sex because he equates lubrication with arousal and enjoyment, she thinks he has "gone off" her because he can't keep an erection. She may begin to think her older body is repulsive, that her partner is having an affair (probably with a woman half her age) and so on, ad infinitum until a minor mechanical problem that could have been solved with a tube of gel from the chemist's shop risks blowing a relationship apart.

Sadly, the negative expectations I've already mentioned may lead both men and women to think that a declining sex life is inevitable and taboos around menopause inherited, perhaps, from their parents' generation, often make it difficult for couples to talk about it.

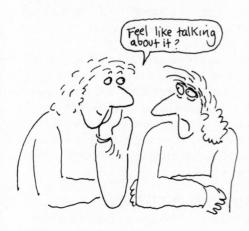

It really is important to talk to your partner, though, if you have any problem with dryness. Firstly, it is important that he knows it does not signal any lack of response on your part. Because young women usually secrete vaginal fluids as soon as they are aroused it's easy to equate the two. Secondly, your partner needs to know that longer foreplay may be all that is needed – many older women just need more time for their lubricating glands to work – and finally you both need to know that if that is not enough, there are simple solutions to the problem.

In referring to a partner as "he" I am not overlooking lesbian partnerships, but assuming that a woman is more likely to understand the changes in her lover's body. However, if there is a big age difference the younger woman may not be aware of every aspect of menopause, so talking about it is again important.

The orthodox approach is to give HRT or creams containing oestrogen to be applied locally. These creams deliver oestrogen directly to the walls of the vagina and are much safer than HRT but even so a small amount of oestrogen gets into the bloodstream. If you'd rather avoid that, an aromatherapist or medical herbalist can make you a cream containing plant oestrogens that have a similar effect with less risks or you can make it up yourself (see Appendix A). Such creams are not intended to be used as lubricants during intercourse but used at other times. Simple lubricants such as creams, gels, saliva (or even sour cream!) are the most straightforward answer.

The really good news, though, is that making love often and having plenty of orgasms is the best way to keep vaginal dryness at bay. A lot of books about menopause refer to "frequent intercourse" preventing dryness but it is important to understand that it is not penetration that keeps the lubricating glands active, but the process of arousal, enjoyment and orgasm. In other words, lovemaking between two women, masturbation or non-penetrative sex with a male partner will have the same effect.

The pelvic floor exercises described in Chapter 17 help to prevent dryness because they improve circulation in the genital area, and any part of your body will function best when it has a rich blood supply. Strengthening your pelvic muscles can increase pleasure in other ways, too. Some women who had not been able to reach orgasm find that they can after doing these exercises for a while and if you are in a heterosexual relationship, try using your pelvic muscles to gently squeeze your partner's penis.

SEXUALLY TRANSMITTED DISEASES

Don't kid yourself that these things don't happen to older women!

Listen to this story from A. who understandably wants to remain anonymous:

"I was 57 and divorced ten years when I met Jack, and I'd been on my own for most of that time. We hit it off immediately and after a while we became lovers. He was working in London and stayed there four or five nights a week but we spent all our weekends together. Our love-life was very good, and often quite energetic! I had no problem with dryness but I did sometimes tear a little around my vagina. I hadn't menstruated for about eight years at that point, and I suppose the skin was thinning a bit. One weekend he said he wouldn't sleep with me because he had a sore on his penis. He used to joke that he needed a girl-friend in London for weekdays and me in Berkshire for weekends. I began to suspect that it was more than a joke and he eventually admitted that was true. In brief, we had a flaming row and split up. Once people knew we were no longer together they began to tell me about his earlier promiscuity 'You looked so happy I didn't like to say anything before' one friend commented.

I took myself off to hospital and got tested for gonorrhoea, non-specific urethritis and syphilis which were all negative, but Aids was the thing that was worrying me most because of the tears I'd had. I knew that the HIV virus enters the body through broken skin and that it was increasing among heterosexuals. The hospital would not test for HIV because it was too soon for any antibodies to show up, but when I asked if I could come back in three or four months' time, they counselled me not to have the test unless I wanted to enter another relationship. It preyed on my mind for a year and eventually I went back and fibbed about having a new fiancé so I could get tested. The test was negative, but I'd spent a whole year worrying about it. If I meet anybody else I want to get close to, I shall remember everything I've ever read about safe sex!"

A. is correct, of course, in saying that the HIV virus enters the body through broken skin, but any infection will do so more easily than through skin that is whole: herpes, gonorrhoea, syphilis, NSU as well as HIV. If the walls of your vagina are dry or thinning you need to be even more careful when entering a new relationship. Use a condom, or stick to non-penetrative sex. (When using condoms, remember not to use any oil or oil-based lubricant at the same time, as these attack and quite quickly break down rubber. For safety, use a gel designed for this purpose.) Yes, it is a nuisance having to think about such things just when you've stopped worrying about getting pregnant, but far better than risking infections that range from unpleasant to life-threatening.

CONTRACEPTION

During the peri-menopause (the time leading up to the end of menstruation) it is still possible to become pregnant and if periods are irregular the beginning of a pregnancy might be mistaken for just another gap between periods. If you have been using a natural method of fertility awareness, based on temperature changes and the state of the vaginal mucus, it may become harder to be sure when you are fertile as ovulation becomes less regular. At this time, too, less mucus may be produced which distorts the reading. You might decide to use a barrier method (condoms or diaphragm) for a while.

Whichever form of contraception you choose, it is important to go on using it until a year after your last period. American Indian women count thirteen full moons after their last menstruation (there are thirteen lunar months in one calendar year) and celebrate their new status as a post-menopausal women on the fourteenth full moon. Orthodox western medicine may be less poetic, but is in agreement on the timing.

RELATIONSHIPS AT MID-LIFE

So far, I've written mostly about the mechanics of sex. Discussing love and relationships at mid-life and after is more problematical because the way human beings interact is as varied, complex and individual now as at any other time. People fall in and out of love, marry, divorce, remarry, are faithful or not, or remain celibate by choice or through circumstances.

When couples break up at mid-life, the reasons seldom lie with the physical events of menopause. I've already stressed the importance of talking to your partner about any physical problems, and couples who communicate well with each other are unlikely to be affected by the changes in a woman's body. Where communication is not good, stresses have often built up over a long time and there are usually problems in the relationship that have nothing to do with menopause. Couples who have stuck together unhappily "for the sake of the children" often break up when the children become independent, and for many women this happens to coincide with menopause.

Menopause may be used as a smokescreen to obscure the real problems facing a couple. Because menopausal women are popularly imagined to be neurotic, some men blame their partner's unhappiness on "the change". It can be a handy excuse for anything that is not going well between them. A woman may also convince herself that she feels tense, anxious and unhappy because she's perimenopausal: it's reassuring to have a physical explanation for her misery and it sidesteps looking at the true issues.

Women also blame their physical changes, particularly any signs of aging in their bodies, if their partners leave them for another woman – especially if she is younger – though where the relationship is secure in other respects it is very unlikely that the first grey hairs or a few extra pounds in weight would be enough to break it.

Men have their own difficulties at mid-life, which coincide with their partner's menopause. They may feel as threatened by the first signs of aging as she is, they may have financial problems or face difficult decisions about their career, all of which have repercussions within the relationship. Again, if a couple are able to talk constructively they are likely to come through such a stressful period without threat to their future together.

When couples have difficulty communicating, counselling can help. A trained counsellor will usually listen to each partner separately before arranging some sessions for both together. This allows each person to put forward their perception of the relationship, why it is not working and what the problems are, without acrimony and without interruption before coming together with the counsellor as mediator. Joint sessions allow the couple to explore ways in which they can overcome their differences. If the relationship has deteriorated to the point where it is beyond saving, counselling sessions can often help partners to separate with less emotional damage.

If you are having relationship problems, do please think about the possibility of counselling. Even if your partner refuses to see a counsellor with you, individual sessions can help you survive a traumatic time and move forward in life with a better understanding of your own emotional needs and responses. If you are divorced, or have come out of a long-term relationship, even if it was some time ago, you may find counselling helps you to resolve old hurts and be more able to form a successful new partnership, if that is what you would like, or to enjoy your life as a single, independent woman.

Moving on beyond mid-life, whether you are in an established relationship, or a relatively new one, or on your own, the future is not a loveless, sexless desert.

Marguerite Duras, the French novelist makes no secret of her relationship with her lover who is 36. In fact her latest book, written at 78, is a chronicle of their love. " Ah yes, but she's French" I hear you thinking! But here is her English contemporary, Mary Wesley: "People seem to think that you don't know anything about sex after your're 40 or 50. That's ridiculous. You know a great deal more about sex when you're 80 than when you're 40".

To that I would add that you know a great deal more about love, too. Falling in love at 60 is just as tumultuous, wonderful or painful as at 16, but you have so much more experience behind you to help you understand both your own feelings and those of your partner. Still being in love at 70 with the person you loved at 17 is a very blessed state. Whether your future involves developing a new relationship or deepening an old one, the years from mid-life onwards can be emotionally rich and rewarding.

PART II
TAKING CARE OF YOURSELF

Do you know how to get the best out of your doctor? Where to look for help if you don't want to take drugs? What kind of exercise strengthens your bones? Or which foods protect you from cancer?

Do you want to keep your brain active into old age? And your love-life?

This part of the book will tell you how.

8

GETTING THE BEST
FROM YOUR DOCTOR

FREEDOM TO MAKE choices is one aspect of personal power, and a sense of powerlessness and frustration is something that many women experience when looking for professional help with discomforts or more serious physical problems during menopause. A major concern, which I have heard voiced over and over again, is that the medical profession seems to have polarised into two extremes: at one end, the doctors who advocate hormone replacement therapy as the only possible treatment for even minor ills, and at the other, those who offer no help beyond the advice to "Grin and bear it".

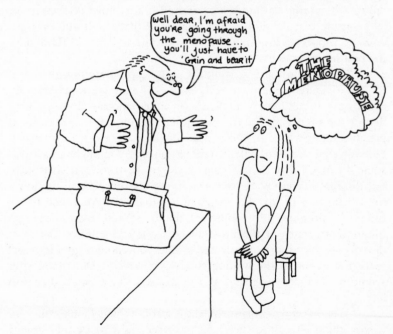

It is easy to lay all the blame for this state of affairs on the medical profession as a whole, or on individual doctors, but we, as women, have to take our share of responsibility. Too often, women feel that their problems are "not worth bothering about" and if they consult a doctor at all, do so in an almost apologetic manner. If we do not take our own health seriously, how can we expect our doctors to do so?

Another prevalent, and potentially dangerous, notion is that any health problems experienced by women between about 40 and 50 is caused by "the change", particularly pain in the abdominal area. "Well, at your age, what can you expect?" is a common response and one that, sadly, one hears from doctors and patients alike. But NO PART OF THE NORMAL PROCESS OF MENOPAUSE IS PAINFUL and you should never blame the menopause for any pain, unusual symptom or anything that simply doesn't "feel right". This can lead to the first signs of various cancers and other serious disease being overlooked until it is too late for effective treatment.

Any worrying symptom should be investigated, whatever your age. I hope that Chapter 2 has given you an idea of what is "normal", so you can judge for yourself if anything you experience falls outside that definition. Just remember that any health problem deserves proper attention, whatever your age, and that YOU deserve the best health possible.

One step towards getting the most appropriate health care is to get to know your own body well. Do you know where your ovaries are located? or your liver? or your pancreas? It helps your doctor (or alternative health practitioner) if you can be as precise as possible about where you have pain, discomfort or other symptoms. Nobody expects you to talk medical jargon, and you might antagonise some doctors if they think you are trying to be too clever! It is helpful, though, if you say "I have a dull, continuous ache in the lower right-hand side of my abdomen" rather than "I have a pain in my tummy". Although any competent doctor should ask you enough questions to pinpoint the problem area, the sad truth is that most doctors are very short of time and asking you enough questions will make the queue in the waiting room even longer. Describing your symptoms accurately will help your doctor to make a correct diagnosis faster.

Whether a particular problem is attributable to menopause, or is something else altogether, you have the right to be told exactly what is wrong, what the proposed treatment is, whether there are any side-effects and whether there is any other possible treatment available. Ask as many questions as you need to establish all the facts before you make a decision. The "Patient's Charter" states that you have the right "To be given a clear explanation of any treatment proposed, including any risks and any alternatives, before you decide whether you will agree to the treatment."

Unfortunately, answering questions takes even longer than asking them, and a doctor pressed for time may not go into as much detail as you want. If so, ask for a return appointment to thoroughly clarify any points that have not been covered in your initial visit, or find out whether there is a Well Woman Clinic or Menopause Clinic in your area, where you are likely to be allocated more time.

There are, of course, excellent doctors who will take time to discuss all the options with you and tell you about the drawbacks as well as the benefits of any proposed treatment, but women's experiences suggest that they are in a minority.

You also have a right to refuse medical treatment, if you so wish. A doctor who tells you that you "have to" have a hysterectomy, or take replacement hormones, or whatever, is only expressing an opinion, and cannot force you to do so against your will.

Not all doctors in general practice are as well informed as they might be about handling menopause. In particular, there is still much misunderstanding of hormone replacement, especially among older doctors who graduated from medical school before HRT was widely used. I have heard of doctors prescribing HRT for women who were experiencing only very minor difficulties with their menopause or even no symptoms at all. Worse still, giving replacement hormones as a preventive measure for women approaching menopause. (At that point, there is not yet any drop in hormone levels, so there is no need for "replacement".) Unfortunately, the women involved thought this was wonderful! "I simply can't afford to have a menopause" one high-powered lady told me. I doubt very much if they would have thought this was so marvellous if the treatment had been fully explained to them. If you want to try this form of therapy, ask to be told about possible side-effects, both long and short term, and if you are worried about any of these, enquire about the possibility of other approaches. Several drugs have been developed in recent years which appear to present a viable alternative to hormones.

If you are not happy about the prospect of taking hormones or drugs for ten to fifteen years or even longer, this really leaves you with no choice at all unless you look beyond mainstream medicine at some of the alternative or complementary therapies.

Theoretically, it is possible for your doctor to offer any of these therapies within the framework of the National Health Service, but in reality this option is not often available. Only a minority of doctors are both well-informed about, and sympathetic towards the wide range of other therapies, and those that are seldom have the funds to offer them to patients.

You can only choose wisely when you have all the facts so in the following chapter you will find brief reviews of various therapies so that you have enough information to make informed choices about your own health and well-being.

FURTHER READING:

Our Bodies Ourselves	Ed. Phillips & Rakusen	*Penguin*
The Anatomy Colouring Book	Kapit & Elson	*Harper & Row*

9

WIDENING YOUR CHOICES

As I suggested at the end of the last chapter, you might find one or more of the following therapies a viable alternative to the orthodox medical approach, or a valuable complement to medical treatment.

As well as discussing how practitioners of various therapies might be able to help you, I have indicated where it is possible to draw on these systems to help yourself, because knowing what you can do to help yourself is perhaps the most empowering choice of all.

ACUPUNCTURE AND ACUPRESSURE

Acupuncture is part of Traditional Chinese Medicine (TCM) although in the West the part is better-known than the whole. TCM itself is part of a wider spectrum of Oriental medicine which includes Shiatsu, Reiki, Shen Tao (acupressure), Qui Gong and the martial arts all of which are forms of energy medicine. Energy medicine is abaout maintaining ones health and well-being. Whether a practitioner uses acupuncture alone, or includes Chinese herbs, dietary advice, etc., the aim is to balance the energy, or life-force, known as Chi or Qi, flowing through our bodies. This energy can take two forms: Yin, which is cold, moist, dark, passive and Yang, which is hot, dry, light and active. For perfect health, we need to have both in balance. This balance is not a passive state, but a kind of dynamic equilibrium which is constantly changing.

This balance of energies is affected by many factors, including the time of year and even the time of day. An important concept is that of the Five Elements: Fire, Earth, Metal, Water and Wood. These don't refer to the physical materials, metal, wood and so forth, but to the kind of energy that they represent. Each of the major organs in the body is governed by one of these elements and they all interact with each other.

Chi flows through our bodies via a system of pathways called meridians, the Yin energy moving upwards in the meridians at the front of the body and the Yang energy moving downwards through those at the back. Each meridian governs a major organ or body system and they are linked in pairs, each pair consisting of one Yin and one Yang meridian. There are also connections linking all of the pathways to each other. When Chi is flowing freely and evenly throughout the body we experience good health but when, for any reason, it is unable to flow freely, there may be too much energy in some parts of the body and too little in others, and then patterns of dis-ease may appear. The acupuncturist's aim is to maintain or restore good health by balancing the flow. This is done by inserting very fine needles at specific points on the meridians.

At a first consultation, the acupuncturist will take a very long and detailed history of your health and lifestyle, as well as your current health problems. This will give him or her an overall picture of your personal Chi. He/she will then feel your pulses – six in each wrist – which complete the picture by showing how your energies are at that moment. On the basis of all this information he/she will then decide where to place the needles.

The needles are ultra-fine, some no more than a hair's width, and do not cause pain. At most, there is slight temporary discomfort but often a needle can be inserted without the patient feeling it at all. One the needle is in place, the patient may feel some odd sensations, such as tingling, pressure, etc. and these tell the therapist what effect the needles are having on the energy in the meridians. He/she may sometimes wiggle a needle to increase its effect.

Because of the risk of infection from shared needles, most acupuncturists now use disposable needles or, if you are being treated on a regular or long-term basis, may keep a set of needles used only for you and sterilised between visits.

Most acupuncturists also use moxa, a dried herb which is burnt to produce warmth. This is done particularly if the body is lacking hot, dry energy. Either a small twist of moxa is placed on top of a needle that is already in place and lit, or the therapist will light a cigar-like stick of moxa and hold it over the areas of the body that need more heat. The effect is very comforting.

Acupressure, or Shen Tao, shares the same underlying theory and philosophy as Acupuncture. It is sometimes called "Acupuncture without needles" and as the term implies, the therapy involves applying pressure to meridian points to influence the energy, or Chi, flowing through the body.

A consultation will follow the same pattern as for Acupuncture and the practitioner will feel the pulses in both your wrists before deciding which meridian points to treat. This is usually done via a series of holds, using both hands to press gently on two points at a time. The treatment is gentle and extremely relaxing. It is not unknown for the patient to fall asleep on the couch!

(See also entry for Traditional Chinese Medicine)

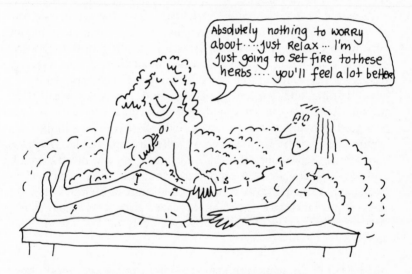

SELF-HELP: DIY acupuncture is well-nigh impossible! You could apply pressure to some of your own meridian points to alleviate symptoms such as hot flushes. Get a well-illustrated book or ask a qualified practitioner to show you where and how to press.

ALEXANDER TECHNIQUE

The Alexander Technique is concerned with the way we use all our senses and how we move our bodies: how we stand, walk, sit, get up from a chair and so forth. Poor use of our senses, including in-appropriate use of our bodies underlie many problems that arise in our middle years and later, when bad habits that may not have affected our health when we were younger, begin to take their toll. Back pain is an obvious example but many other conditions are helped by improving the use of our senses and body movement.

An Alexander teacher will begin by looking carefully at the way you walk, sit, stand etc., and then gently make you aware of anything you are doing that is detrimental to your self. This is most often done by gentle touch and guiding you in movement in a slightly different way, becoming aware of various muscle groups, or allowing a different part of your body to "lead" the movement. To start with, the sessions will probably concentrate on the basic movements I've already mentioned, but you can also ask the teacher to help you find the best way of carrying out any special activity that you do regularly, such as the best way to sit at your desk, drive the car or play the violin. The process of re-educating your self can be quite lengthy but very rewarding. People who try Alexander work almost always experience a reduction of stress, increased mental clarity and a greater feeling of well-being, as well as reducing physical aches and pains.

During and after menopause, good posture is particularly important. If you can stand and walk in balance you will not only look younger and stay far more mobile than your slouching contemporaries, but be far less likely to suffer from backache. Balanced posture can help reduce the chance of prolapse, because the womb and other organs are well supported within the pelvic girdle when you stand in balance. Your lungs function more efficiently if they are not cramped inside a slumping rib-cage. Even your brain works better when your head rests easily and freely on the top of your spine!

SELF-HELP: Difficult, although there are one or two good books which describe exercises and ways of applying Alexander's principles in your daily activities. If you can't afford a lengthy series of lessons, try to invest in at least a few sessions with a teacher before working from a book.

AROMATHERAPY

Aromatherapy makes use of essential oils extracted from plants to increase health and well-being. These oils are very concentrated and must always be diluted before use. They are also very complex, each one containing many different compounds from the plant, sometimes as many as 300 in one oil.

The main use of the oils is in massage, though they are also used in baths, compresses, vapourisers, inhalations and in creams for skin treatment. If you consult an aromatherapist, you will almost certainly be offered massage during the visit and the therapist may well give you oils to take away for use in baths, etc.

Essential oils can help a wide variety of physical, mental and emotional conditions and aromatherapists take a holistic view of their clients rather than symptom-treating. It is also a wonderful form of preventive health-care: giving yourself time to enjoy a massage with beautifully scented oil really does reduce stress which underlies so much illness. Aromatherapy also helps a wide range of physical problems.

During menopause an aromatherapist may use oils such as Geranium which balance hormone production, Cypress to help control heavy bleeding, Sage or Clary Sage which contain oestrogen-like substances (plant oestrogens) to help maintain your own oestrogen levels, Rosemary to support your adrenal glands and Rose or Jasmine to strengthen your whole reproductive system. Other oils will be chosen according to your particular needs: the therapist will want to know if you are feeling stressed, tired, depressed, anxious, if you have any aches and pains, and so forth. On the basis of all this information he or she will make a blend of oils that correspond to your physical, mental and emotional needs at that moment. At future visits, the blend may be quite different as your needs change.

SELF-HELP: You can benefit a great deal from using essential oils in your bath, in vapourisers (burners), as a personal perfume or in simple self-massage. Remember that essential oils are very concentrated and must always be diluted before use. 3 drops of essential oil to 5 mls of a vegetable oil such as almond, grapeseed, sunflower or soya oil is the safe dilution for massage. For baths, add 6 drops of oil after running the bath and just before you get into it.

Look for an introductory weekend workshop where you can learn the basics, or check on the safe use of oils from a book.

You will find more details of oils for specific problems in the next chapter and in Appendix A.

BACH FLOWER REMEDIES

The flower remedies developed by Dr. Edward Bach act upon the mental, emotional and spiritual levels. The intent is to help transform negative mental states into positive ones, but because we cannot divorce our bodies from our minds and souls, physical health often improves when the remedies are used.

The remedies are prepared by infusing the flowers of various plants, trees and shrubs in pure springwater. Brandy is added to the water to act as a preservative, and three or four drops of the resulting remedy is added to a glass of water or placed on the tongue, when needed. The remedies are so dilute as to be akin to homoeopathy (Dr. Bach was a homoeopath before he developed this system of healing).

The most important Flower Remedy for menopausal women is Walnut. Walnut offers support in any time of change or transition, whether it be adolescence, a change of job, divorce or moving house and the menopause is no exception. The choice of other remedies will depend very much on your personality and how you react to different situations. It will also vary from time to time as your moods and circumstances alter.

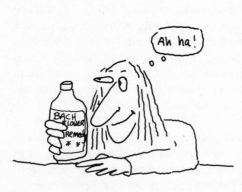

The Remedies are more often used in blends than singly, so a blend to help you during menopause is likely to include Walnut, one remedy that corresponds to your underlying personality and one or two others indicated by your immediate needs. For example, if you feel fearful about the menopause or post-menopausal years because you do not know what to expect from them, Aspen might be included, but if you fear something specific, then Mimulus would be more appropriate. Mustard is helpful in some forms of depression and Gentian, Gorse or Sweet Chestnut for others. Beyond this, it is impossible to give specific advice in a book, as there are 38 Remedies, which can be combined in infinite variations and even the right combination for you might not be the same two days running!

SELF-HELP: The Bach Remedies are ideally suited to self-help. They are totally safe in use and if you should choose the "wrong" one, it will simply have no effect on you. It was always Dr. Bach's intention that they should be available for use by lay people. You might like to attend a seminar on the Remedies, or you can use books to help you decide on the most suitable remedy. If you are familiar with the techniques of dowsing, this is a very good way of selecting the most helpful Remedy. Whichever Remedies you select for yourself, include some Walnut in the blend. Only make up enough to last you for a few days, or a week at the most, then review the situation as your needs may change quite quickly.

COUNSELLING AND PSYCHOTHERAPY

Counselling and psychotherapy can be valuable ways of dealing with the depression, anxiety and other emotional problems that arise in mid-life. These are often blamed on the physical menopause – indeed the neurotic menopausal woman has become a stereotype – but apart from a tendency to feel more emotional at times when hormone levels are fluctuating (such as in adolescence, pregnancy or pre-menstrually, as well as during the menopause) there is really no connection. Rather, the physical changes happen to coincide with a time of life when stressful or emotionally disturbing situations are likely to arise: from children leaving home to career difficulties, problems within a marriage or financial worries. When we are passing through our own mid-life transition is often the time when our parents die, and talking to somebody who is experienced in bereavement counselling can be a great help.

I have grouped these therapies together here because the dividing line between counselling and psychotherapy is a rather wobbly one! To complicate matters, some psychotherapists call themselves counsellors because of the widely-held misconception that anybody needing psychotherapy must be mentally ill. Sadly, this can stop people who would really benefit from such help from asking for it. Thousands of completely sane and otherwise well-balanced people have found psychotherapy a profound help in understanding and recovering from a period of depression or some particularly distressing event in their life, and often feel that their time in therapy has been a period of great personal growth.

Talking to a trained counsellor or psychotherapist is often more effective than the antidepressants and other drugs often prescribed to help mental or emotional stress and of course there is no danger of side effects or addiction. There are many different approaches to counselling and a variety of systems of psychotherapy

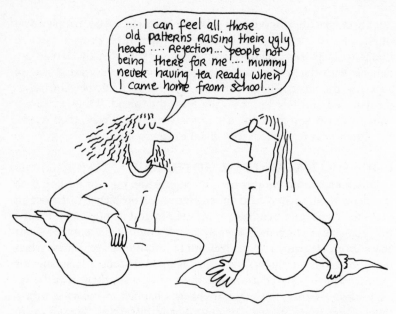

and this is, of course, an area where the therapists's personality is an important factor, so it is possible that the first person you see may not feel like the right one to help you. Therapists themselves are well aware of this and will usually offer you one exploratory consultation before you commit yourself to further sessions. Once you are happy with your choice of a counsellor, he or she may ask you to make a commitment to a minimum of, say, six sessions. This is because you are unlikely to get any lasting benefit from just one or two.

Most counsellors practise privately, but in many areas you will find voluntary organisations offering free or low-cost counselling services. Relate (formerly the Marriage Guidance Council) offers counselling for couples experiencing difficulties in their relationship. Cruse provides access to trained bereavement counsellors and your doctor's surgery or the Citizen's Advice Bureau should have addresses of these and other organizations offering more general counselling. Some forms of psychotherapy are available through the National Health Service, but there are often very long waiting lists which mean that you may not be able to get help when you need it most and patients have no choice as to which therapist they will see. Most psychotherapists practise privately, often through natural health centres or clinics.

If you are bewildered by the great variety of psychotherapeutic approaches on offer, talk to one or two therapists to find out what their work involves. Is it a simple "talking therapy" or do they include movement, art-work, role-play, visualization, etc.? The right one for you will depend very much on your temperament and personality.

SELF-HELP: You might try talking to a trusted friend but it is often easier and more effective to talk to a trained therapist who is not in any way involved in your issues and will probably have met many other people before you in similar situations. To know that your problems are neither unique nor abnormal, but shared by many others, can be a great comfort.

CRANIOSACRAL THERAPY
(sometimes called CRANIAL OSTEOPATHY)

Craniosacral therapy aims to help the body in its own healing and balancing processes. It focuses on what is called the cranio-sacral mechanism, a rhythmic impulse arising in the central nervous system which can be felt throughout the body. Any restrictions to this pulse can have repercussions on our wellbeing at every level – mental, physical and emotional. The rhythm can be affected by blows, falls, accidents (whether they took place recently or a long time ago) a difficult labour or even difficulty at the time of your own birth but they may equally be due to mental attitudes.

The therapist uses extremely gentle and subtle touch to identify and correct whatever is disrupting this rhythm. This is done by means of various holds applied to the head, hips, sacrum, spine or various parts of the body. The amount of pressure used is so light as to be barely perceptible, but the results are very powerful. After a treatment you will probably feel extremely relaxed, even drowsy, but this can be followed by a state of great mental clarity, in addition to relief from a great variety of physical problems.

Craniosacral therapists sometimes describe what they do as "listening with their hands". Your body tells its own story through the subtle rhythms and patterns that the therapist can feel, making this a very personal and individualised form of therapy.

Craniosacral therapy is valuable during any time of change, helping you to adjust to a new way of being. During menopause more specifically, the therapist will use gentle touch on your head to identify and release any tensions and restrictions that affect the proper functioning of the Pituitary Gland. This is the "master gland" that regulates all hormone production so ensuring that it functions normally is important at this time when many symptoms, such as hot flushes, are directly caused by fluctuating hormone levels.

Depression, which may be experienced at mid-life, is often helped by craniosacral therapy, both by easing tensions in the physical body and through the caring, listening approach of the therapist. Clients often find their physical vitality increases as their depression lifts.

SELF-HELP: Not possible.

DIETARY THERAPY

What you eat can profoundly influence your health, for good or bad, and relatively simple changes in diet have brought relief from pre-menstrual syndrome and menopausal problems for thousands of women. Sorting out which foods, combinations of foods, supplements, cooking methods etc., are the best for you can be very confusing, though, especially as there are a variety of approaches. You may well get advice on these ares from a medical herbalist, acupuncturist, naturopath, homoeopath, Doctor of Chinese Medicine or other practitioner as part of their overall approach to improving your health. Otherwise, you can get help from a nutritional counsellor. Look for somebody trained by the Institute of Optimum Nutrition or the Green Farm Nutrition Centre or write to The Women's Nutritional Advisory Service which specialises in advice on foods for women suffering from pre-menstrual syndrome or menopausal problems. You can find addresses for all these organisations at the end of this book.

SELF-HELP: If you follow the nutritional advice in this book you can't go too far wrong. To expand on it, there are plenty of books on healthy eating, often with recipes and cooking methods.

HEALING

To define and describe healing is not easy, partly because there are as many ways of healing as there are healers and partly because nobody can really say how healing "works". However, all the healers I have talked with agree that they act as channels for a healing energy which flows through them.

Many healers place their hands on the body of the person

seeking healing, either on the head, or on the part of the body that needs help, or both. Others work with their hands a little distance from body to influence the aura, or subtle body. Many healers combine both these approaches.

Many people who practise "hands on" therapies of various kinds, such as reflexology, massage, aromatherapy, craniosacral therapy, etc., undoubtedly transmit healing energy through their hands, but few of them would describe themselves as healers. This term is usually reserved for those who work with healing energy outside of any specific system. However, there are also forms of healing that do use various methods to enhance or focus the transmission of healing energy. These include colour healing, crystal healing and the use of sound.

Healing can be experienced at every level: physical, mental, emotional and spiritual. Virtually any physical disease can be helped through healing, as well as deeply-held emotional trauma. Although it is true that physical illness is often helped or totally eliminated, healing should not be equated with "curing". The greatest healing for some people may come from seeing that their illness is an opportunity for learning. For a terminally ill person, healing might mean being enabled to approach death peacefully, even joyously.

It might not have occurred to you to ask a healer for help with mid-life problems, but in fact healing can relieve stress, insomnia, depression and other physical and emotional problems and help your body and mind to adjust to change.

The majority of healers in Great Britain are members of the National Federation of Spiritual Healers, but this does not mean that a non-member cannot be a fine healer. The Federation keeps a register of members and can put you in touch with healers in your area. Otherwise you can go by personal recommendation.

SELF-HELP: Self-healing is possible, often by using meditation or visualization techniques. You may be able to find workshops on self-healing in some areas, otherwise a simple method is to sit quietly and imagine the area of pain or dis-ease bathed in gold (or white) light, then see the light washing away all pain and sickness and bringing in healing energy.

HERBAL MEDICINE
Plants were the first medicines known to humans, and modern herbal medicine is part of an unbroken tradition that stretches back into

pre-history. We know something of the plants that our earliest ancestors used because archaeologists have been able to identify plant remains found in early burial places and living sites. Apart from the food plants, nearly all these remains are of plants which we know to be medicinal.

The "building blocks" from which plant cells are made are the same as those from which the cells of the human body are formed, so the medical herbalist can select plants that bring into our bodies various elements that we need for our health.

Sometimes the whole plant is used, or part of the plant such as the leaves, flowers, seeds or roots is chosen, often because that part contains the largest amounts of the active compounds. The plant material may be used fresh or dried but is more often made into extracts and tinctures. These enable the herbalist to use the most appropriate plant at any time, without being dependent on the growing season of the plant. It also makes it possible to use plants from all parts of the world. Dried plant material can also be made into infusions "or "teas") or powdered and put into capsules or compressed into tablet form. Extracts or tinctures are mixed into creams for treating skin conditions.

Like most natural health practitioners, a medical herbalist will take a long and detailed history of your health at the first consultation before deciding on the best plants to help your immediate problem. Many herbalists also give advice on diet and lifestyle and treatment will be designed to benefit the whole person, not a set of symptoms.

Herbs which are particularly helpful during and after menopause are those which contain plant compounds similar to human hormones. These may provide the body with elements it needs for its own production of hormones, or may have a similar effect on the body to that of human hormones. Chasteberry is a particularly valuable example, as it normalises production of oestrogen and progesterone. A number of plants contain compounds resembling oestrogen and are often referred to as "plant oestrogens". Although purists may tell you that there is no such thing, the term is a useful shorthand used widely by herbalists and others, so I shall use it in this sense. Oestrogen plants include Fennel, Sage, Liquorice and False Unicorn Root.

A herbalist may also help you with plants that strengthen the reproductive organs or support the adrenal glands which have an important role, as they continue to make some oestrogen after the ovaries stop doing so. Herbs for the adrenals include Borage, Ginseng and Wild Yam, as well as Liquorice which I have already mentioned. These are particularly important if you are experiencing a lot of stress or have had long periods of stress in the past, as this can leave the adrenals very depleted. The same is true if you have been on steroids at any time. These drugs place a great deal of strain on the adrenal glands and this can interfere with their functioning which is so important in the post-menopausal years

SELF-HELP: You can safely use herb teas or infusions such as Liquorice, Fennel, etc. on a daily basis to maintain good health as these are very gentle but effective in their action. You will find directions for some more complex formulae for specific problems in Appendix A. You might also use herbal capsules or tablets from health-food shops but if you have any serious or persistent problem, do consult a qualified medical herbalist for advice.

HOMOEOPATHY

Homoeopathy is sometimes described as "the magic of the minimum dose" and also as "like curing like". A homoeopathic remedy is prepared by taking a substance that can cause certain symptoms and diluting it, then diluting the dilution and so on, sometimes as much as a thousand times. This material may be of plant, mineral or animal origin. At each dilution, the remedy is shaken or "succussed". The remedy is then used to treat conditions with symptoms similar to that which the original substance can cause.

These remedies do not work in the same way as a herbal remedy or synthetic drug, both of which have a measurable effect on the chemistry of our bodies, because by the time all these dilutions have been carried out, it is impossible to detect any of the original material from which the remedy was prepared. The remedies work in a far more subtle way, and can be thought of as carrying something of the energy of that original material. The process of succussion is thought to somehow leave an energy "imprint" in the water/alcohol solution so that when the original material is all gone, the energy pattern remains. The more the remedy has been diluted and succussed, the more active or potent it seems to be, so the various dilutions are called "potentisations". A simple way of explaining what homoeopathy does is that it gives a "jump start" to the body's own ability to heal.

Homoeopathy is a truly holistic therapy in that the practitioner takes into account every facet of the patient's being: physique, personality, lifestyle, even their preferences for different foods and how they feel in different weather conditions. At a first consultation with a homoeopath you may feel that some of the questions you are asked are completely irrelevant to the problem for which you are seeking help, but your answers will help guide the homoeopath to the precise remedy that is right for you. The next patient may have exactly the same symptoms but be prescribed a different remedy because other factors in their life are different. In other words, the homoeopath treats the whole person, not the symptoms.

If the homoeopath decides to use a very high potency remedy, perhaps a 1,000 potentisation, he or she will give you a single dose during your visit, and ask you to come back in a week, two weeks or more to assess what effect it has had. If a low potency seems more appropriate, you may be given tiny tablets to take three or four times a day. While using homoeopathic remedies you will probably be asked to avoid tea, coffee, strongly flavoured foods and to keep your remedy stored away from strong smells.

Homoeopaths believe that the degree to which a woman experiences menopausal symptoms such as hot flushes, sleeplessness, anxiety or heavy bleeding depends on the underlying strength or weakness of her constitution so any homoeopathic remedy may be required to treat the underlying condition and if professional help is sought it is possible to give long term help. However, a few specific remedies crop up repeatedly which can relieve symptoms, though not necessarily cure them. The most common of these are Lachesis, Pulsatilla, Sepia, Sulphur and Calc-carb. The first three of these are often needed at times of great hormone change: puberty and pregnancy, as well as menopause.

If you are thinking about consulting a homoeopath it is better, if possible, to do so before taking HRT, so that the homoeopath has a clear picture of your symptoms rather than the changes brought about by the hormone treatment.

While most homoeopaths practise privately, it is easier to have access to homoeopathy through the National Health Service than virtually any other alternative therapy. A few medical doctors are also qualified homoeopaths but you should be aware that some doctors offering homoeopathy have done only a very short training and may be less knowledgeable than a "lay" homoeopath. There are a number of homoeopathic hospitals.

SELF-HELP: You can buy low-potency remedies in some chemists and many health food shops and they can be useful as a form of first-aid for hot flushes, heavy bleeding, etc. However, do read up a bit on homoeopathy before you start self-prescribing and remember that factors other than the obvious symptom may need to be taken into account. If you have any long-term health problem, try to see a qualified homoeopath if you possibly can.

MASSAGE

Massage is one of the oldest, most enjoyable and one of the most effective therapies for reducing mental and emotional stress, muscular tension, and many kinds of pain. Massage can reduce high blood pressure, improve muscle tone, disperse fluid retention, help the appearance of your skin and much more.

The therapist uses a wide variety of strokes, ranging from light stroking to deeper pressure to relax or tone your muscles, stimulate your circulation and lymph system and balance the central nervous system. By varying the strokes, a masseur or masseuse can make the treatment profoundly relaxing or quite invigorating according to the need of the individual client. Some therapists also work on a subtle level to balance the flow of Chi energy (see entries for Shiatsu, etc.) Deep physical relaxation can bring about a lessening of mental and emotional stress.

There are so many different kinds of massage that choosing a therapist can be quite bewildering. If you simply need relief from muscular pain, look for somebody practising Swedish or Remedial Massage, or who specializes in sports injury massage. For a more profoundly relaxing massage which can release mental and emotional, as well as physical, tensions, you might choose between Aroma-therapy, Esalen Massage and Holistic Massage. If you have problems with cellulite or fluid retention, Lymphatic Drainage massage would be more helpful... and so on. If you don't know which kind of massage to choose, talk to the therapist about your needs before booking a session, or act on recommendation from somebody who has had treatment from the therapist you have in mind.

Massage is available at natural health centres, clinics, beauty salons, health clubs, etc. and the location will often give you a good idea of what kind of treatment to expect. Remember that you don't have to have anything "wrong" with you to enjoy a massage! If you possibly can, indulge yourself occasionally or get somebody to treat you to a session as a birthday present.

SELF-HELP: It is possible to massage most areas of your own body, and this is a good second-best if you can't get somebody else to massage you but the one area you really can't reach is your back, and work on the back is probably the most relaxing part of any massage. If you can't get professional massage, try teaming up with a friend to massage each other. You can either learn some simple techniques at a weekend workshop, or use a book or training video.

OSTEOPATHY

Osteopathy is concerned with the body's framework of bones and the muscles, ligaments and other soft tissue that connect them and enable us to move about. Stress, injuries or poor posture can cause pain, loss of mobility and other problems affecting the joints, especially those of the spine. Other factors which lead us to misuse our backs include car driving, poorly-designed furniture, fashion and social pressures so it is not surprising that a great deal of an osteopath's work is concerned with the spine though he or she will also treat injuries or other problems affecting the hips, knees, ankles, shoulders and other joints.

Osteopaths use massage and manipulation to ease pain and to restore movement to joints that are not functioning properly. To assess what the problem is and what treatment will help, the osteopath will feel the muscles, joints and ligaments involved and observe you sitting, standing and lying down as well as bending forwards, sideways and backwards, or turning your head. You will also be asked questions about any pain you feel, when it began, what makes it worse or better and any accidents you may have suffered, recently or longer ago.

Back pain and loss of mobility are increasingly common problems as we grow older and can affect general health, for example by reducing the amount of exercise we can manage, or preventing good quality sleep. An osteopath can help to reduce or minimise the pain and maintain mobility.

Many osteopaths also use cranial osteopathy (see above) and a wide range of manipulative techniques. Most practise privately, often at natural health centres, though there are some clinics attached to the major schools of osteopathy. The General Council and Register of Osteopaths can give you the address of practitioners in you area.

SELF-HELP: Although osteopathy in the strict sense is impossible to practise on yourself, you can help maintain your own mobility and prevent back problems by taking regular, gentle exercise, making sure that your posture is good (see Alexander Technique) and using simple relaxation techniques to avoid muscular tension.

REFLEXOLOGY
(sometimes called REFLEX ZONE THERAPY)

Reflexology is based on the theory that each organ and area of the body is related to a specific area on the feet and can be influenced by pressure on that area (or Zone). A network of invisible pathways connects each organ to its specific point on the foot. These may be compared to the meridian system in Acupuncture and although reflexologists generally state that these are two different systems, the most recent evidence suggests that they may in fact, be the same.

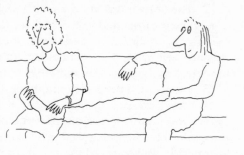

Reflexologists work over the whole of each foot during a treatment, pressing with fingers and thumbs. This enables them to benefit and balance all the body systems at the same time as identifying any area or organ that is not functioning as well as it should, so that they can give extra attention to the reflex points for that area. It is often possible to pick up on weaknesses before they manifest as dis-ease and work on them preventatively.

During menopause, a reflexologist can help you by working on the points relating to the uterus, ovaries, etc., as well as the adrenals which continue to produce oestrogen after the ovaries stop doing so. As I've already suggested, this will be within the framework of a general treatment aimed at balancing and strengthening your whole body. Most people find reflexology very relaxing and regular treatments greatly reduce stress.

SELF-HELP: It is perfectly possible to work on your own feet with the aid of a book and a chart of the reflex points although you lose the benefit of another person's input. This can be a really useful "first-aid" for hot flushes, heavy bleeding, back pain, etc., but you should not view it as an alternative to getting professional advice and treatment and, of course, it is far less relaxing than receiving a treatment from somebody else.

SHIATSU

The name Shiatsu is derived from two Japanese words meaning "finger pressure" and this immediately tells us something about the therapy. Shiatsu practitioners use their fingers and thumbs, but also their elbows, palms of the hands and sometimes even their feet to apply pressure to the meridians at points called tsubos.

The system is based on the same understanding of Chi energy, Yin and Yang as Acupuncture and Traditional Chinese Medicine but has developed in Japan over several centuries. Instead of using needles, Shiatsu uses pressure on the meridian points to influence the flow of Chi, disperse energy blocks and promote good health.

The Shiatsu practitioner knows what kind of energy each pair of meridians carries and will feel where they are overactive and need calming or underactive and need stimulating to rebalance and enhance well-being. Chi energies are not only about physical energy, but relate to the emotions and states of mind, enhancing perception of the 5 senses and deepening intuition.

Regular sessions help to keep us in a state of ease and wellness. Practitioners learn to rebalance our energies which our lifestyles have put out – something that we can all learn to do ourselves. When the energies are well balanced the meridians do not show symptoms and do not get to the stage where illness and dis-ease manifest in our minds or bodies.

Shiatsu practitioners work on the floor, usually on a futon or thick mat. There is no need for the patient to undress, though loose, thinnish clothes are a good idea, as the pressure is applied through the clothing. Practitioners may also manipulate the arms and legs or stretch the whole body. The whole procedure is very relaxing, but you will probably feel quite invigorated afterwards.

Many Shiatsu practitioners include dietary advice, particularly based on Macrobiotics. This system of eating takes into account the way food affects our bodily Chi. Foods are classified according to their Yin or Yang qualities, with meats (very Yang) at one extreme and sugar and very sweet fruits (very Yin) at the other. A balanced diet is made up mainly of grains and vegetables, which fall in the middle of this spectrum, with only small amounts of the extremely Yin or Yang foods. The methods of preparation and cooking also affect the energy of the food and are an important part of the system.

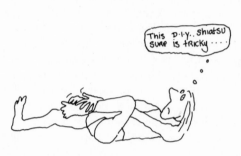

SELF-HELP: You can apply pressure yourself to some of the meridian points but some of them would be difficult or impossible to reach. It would probably be more beneficial to incorporate into your lifestyle some of the other aspects of energy medicine, such as the quality of food, regular meditation and attitude to the environment.

TRADITIONAL CHINESE MEDICINE

Traditional Chinese Medicine (or TCM) embraces acupuncture, Chinese herbs, dietary advice and sometimes breathing exercises (Qi Gong) or other forms of gentle exercise. Everything that I have written above about Acupuncture and Acupressure is equally applicable to TCM and these disciplines are sometimes referred to collectively as Oriental Medicine. The philosophy underlying all forms of Oriental Medicine links us, as human creatures, to the whole of nature: the same laws of energy balance, Yin and Yang, the Five Elements and the succession of the seasons affect the world around us as well as the world within our selves.

TCM differs from the other forms of Oriental medicine mainly in that the practitioner will prescribe herbs as well as using needles or pressure, moxa, etc. to restore balance and health. The herbs may be prescribed in the form of a tincture or pills but many practitioners prefer the traditional method of giving the patient the dried herbs to be boiled and drunk. This is because the actual taste of the herbs – sweet, bitter, sour, etc. has a specific effect on your energy.

The herb Dong Kwai (Chinese Angelica) has attracted much

attention in the West, so much so that you can now buy it in tablet form in many health food stores. It is one of the principal remedies used for menstrual as well as menopausal disturbances, and it is sometimes called "The female Ginseng". Ginseng itself is very valuable during and after menopause because it is an adaptogen, i.e. it helps the body adapt to changing situations. A third remedy, which is very valuable is He Shou Wu. This herb is thought to help prevent osteoporosis, and it also lowers the levels of cholesterol in the blood, so it gives some protection against the two major risks of the post-menopausal years. Traditionally, He Shou Wu was thought to prolong a youthful appearance but it may be that it does so by improving general health and vitality. It is not specific to women but is a generally tonic herb, and older men can benefit from it, too.

These three herbs are all warming in nature, especially Ginseng (which is the most Yang herb). They are all very potent herbs and although they may occasionally be used singly for very short periods of time, traditional practitioners usually prescribe them in a balanced combination with other herbs which prevents or reduces unwanted side-effects. For example Dong Kwai and He Shou Wu both have a laxative effect if used alone, and Ginseng can raise blood-pressure. A person who is very weak may experience palpitations after taking this herb. This does not diminish their very real value, but illustrates why they need to be used carefully.

SELF-HELP: You could very beneficially practise Qui Gong breathing exercises – there are classes and workshops in many areas. It's possible to buy Chinese herbs from specialist importers and even in some Western health food shops, but it's unwise to self-prescribe unless you are well-informed about dosage,timing, etc. Get somebody knowledgeable to advise you if at all possible. If you don't have access to a qualified practitioner but would like to try any of these herbs, it would be wise to do so for a short period only. Try the herbs for a month at most, and see how they affect you.

YOGA

Yoga is, of course, far more than a form of therapy, though there are organisations and individual teachers offering therapeutic or remedial yoga. I include it here because of the tremendous benefits to health that yoga can give at any age. These benefits are not only physical, as yoga is a philosophy as well as a system of exercise, and most classes include periods of relaxation and meditation. Yoga is non-competitive

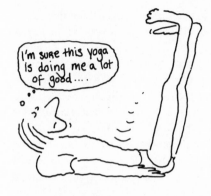

and you will never be asked to do more than your body can safely manage.

The core of any yoga class is the asanas, or postures, each of which is designed to benefit the body and mind in a specific way. Each person in the class can practise these within their own capacity, because the way in which you approach them is more important than achieving a perfect position. Simply trying to do them correctly will give you a great deal of benefit. The teacher will choose a variety of asanas for each lesson which, between them benefit the whole body as well as the mind and spirit.

More specifically, various asanas strengthen different organs of the body, such as the womb, ovaries, adrenals, and practising these really helps the body adjust to the internal changes that take place during menopause.

Almost every local education authority provides yoga classes as part of the adult education programme, and in some places you may also find private teachers. If you look for a teacher who is a member of the British Wheel of Yoga you will know that he or she has been trained to a high standard.

SELF-HELP: There are many books on yoga as well as audio and video cassettes, but there are some drawbacks to teaching yourself. Without a teacher you may not be executing the asanas correctly, in which case you will not get the benefit you expect from them. If at all possible, get some proper tuition first. On the other hand, if you attend a yoga class or have done so in the past and are thoroughly familiar with the postures, there is a great deal to gain from practising regularly at home.

This selection does not comprise every possible alternative therapy: I have, for the most part, concentrated on those therapies which the majority of readers should be able to find fairly easily in their own locality, plus one or two which may need a little more effort in seeking out but which offer particularly valuable help during and after menopause.

If you feel that any of these therapies would benefit you, do look for a practitioner who belongs to the relevant professional body governing his or her discipline. The vast majority of alternative therapists are well trained, ethical and totally professional but unfortunately there is nothing to prevent a person with inadequate training or even no training at all, practising any therapy they choose. Membership of the relevant register is an assurance that your chosen therapist is a bona fides practitioner. Don't be afraid to ask before you make an appointment: the genuine therapist will be only too pleased to tell you his or her qualifications. Or you can write to one of the bodies listed at the back of this book and ask for details of members in your area.

If your income is limited, you may feel that you are denied the choice of any alternative therapy because of the fees involved, but don't be deterred until you have explored the possibility of concessions. Many practitioners work on a sliding scale with lower fees for those who genuinely cannot afford the full cost. If there is a natural health centre or alternative clinic in your area they are quite likely to have a system of concessionary fees. Once again, don't be afraid to ask. Therapists have to earn their living but most of them would rather treat you at a reduced fee than not treat you at all.

FURTHER READING:

Acupuncture	Paul Marcus	*Thorsons*
The Alexander Workbook	Richard Brennan	*Element*
Aromatherapy An A-Z	Patricia Davis	*C.W.Daniel*
Bach Flower Remedies for Woman	Judy Howard	*C.W. Daniel*
Dictionary of the Bach Flower Remedies	T.W. Hyne-Jones	*C.W. Daniel*
Healing Herbs of Edward Bach	J. & M. Barnard	*Bach Educational Prog*
Homoeopathy For The Third Age	Dr. Keith Souter	*C.W. Daniel*
The New Holistic Herbal	D. Hoffmann	*Element*
Natural Healing in Gyneacology	R. Nissim	*Pandora*
Reflexology Today	Doreen Bayly	*Healing Arts Press*
A Woman's Herbal	Kitty Campion	*Vermillion*
Yoga for Women	N. Phelan & M. Volin	*Arrow*

10

HOW TO HELP YOURSELF

A BRIEF GUIDE TO MENOPAUSAL PROBLEMS AND SOLUTIONS.

IN THIS CHAPTER I want to suggest simple ways in which you can help yourself with some of the problems that might arise during menopause. Many of these are suggestions that have come from women who found them valuable during their own menopause. Some are in the nature of "first-aid" which may be all you need in the case of minor discomforts, or which will help until you can see a doctor or other health practitioner. In every instance you should get professional help if your symptoms are severe or persistent.

ANXIETY

Essential oils of Neroli or Ylang Ylang are very helpful. Use them in your bath (6 drops to a bath) regularly and, if possible, get somebody to massage you with them. In an emergency, if you are feeling acutely anxious, simply inhale from the bottle, or from a drop on a tissue.

Breathe in slowly and imagine that as you breathe out you are sending the breath out of the soles of your feet. This is also very helpful for acute anxiety, and doing it regularly can reduce a longer-term problem.

Take Dr. Bach's Rescue Remedy, Aspen, Mimulus, Vervain or other remedies chosen specifically for your needs.

The herb Passiflora (Passiflora incarnata) is effective and you can get it in tablet form at most health-food shops. Other helpful herbs are Valerian (Valeriana officinalis) and Skullcap (Scutellaria laterifolia), which are often found as ingredients in herbal "anti-stress" formulae available in shops. If you prefer you can make your own simple remedy from the dried herbs. Unfortunately, neither of these herbs is very palatable, so if you can obtain them in tincture form, this is an easier way to take them. Use 20 to 30 drops of the tincture in a wineglassful of warm water (with a little honey if you wish) three times a day.

Try to explore what is making your feel anxious by writing your thoughts down, talking with a friend or getting some help from a trained counsellor.

BACK PAIN

Try the back exercises described in "Use it or Lose It". Join a yoga class if at all possible.

Put pain-killing essential oils in your bath: 6 drops of either Camomile or Lavender, or get somebody to massage you with the same oils (3 drops to each 5 mls of vegetable oil) If the problem is purely muscular, this may be all you need. If back pain persists, consult an osteopath.

Alexander technique could be very helpful in the long term.

DEPRESSION

Many essential oils are anti-depressant: Bergamot, Clary Sage, Geranium, Jasmine, Lavender, Rose and Ylang Ylang are probably the most effective. If possible, visit a qualified aromatherapist who will help you discover which is the most helpful for you, as there are many different forms of depression. The support of a trained therapist can be great comfort in depression.

Use one or more of these oils in your bath, as a perfume (just a drop or two on your skin) and in an oil burner in your home.

If you can't get to an aromatherapist, get a friend to massage you.

The Bach Flower Remedies Gentian, Gorse, Mustard, Oak, Olive, Sweet Chestnut, White Chestnut and Wild Rose are each applicable to different types of depression. Consult a Bach practitioner, dowse, use a book to decide which would be the best remedy (or blend of remedies) for you.

Don't bottle up your feelings: talk about them to your friends, partner, children.

Explore the possible reasons for your depression: there may be something simple you can do to remedy them. Get help from a trained counsellor or psychotherapist if your depression persists.

FIBROIDS

Exercises to improve the circulation in the pelvic area: these include sitting cross-legged and rocking from side to side, circling the hips as if swinging a hula-hoop and the exercises described under prolapse.

A detoxifying diet: fresh raw vegetables and fruit, fruit juices and copious amounts of spring water for 3 to 4 days at a time, repeated as often as possible.

Herbs to improve lymphatic drainage: Cleavers, Echinacea, Golden Seal and Poke Root.

Any of these measures helps to stabilize fibroids (prevent them getting any bigger) and in many cases have been shown to reduce the size of fibroids (and therefore the amount of pain or bleeding they cause). They are more effective if used jointly, diet + herbs + exercise.

Acupuncture and homoeopathy have both helped many women.

HEART DISEASE

Use regular exercise and an appropriate diet as preventive measures, see "Use It or Lose It" and "Fuel for Life" for details.

The herbal remedy Hawthorn helps high blood pressure, also fresh, raw garlic. If possible, consult a medical herbalist before using them: otherwise, use for a short time only and see your doctor.

HEAVY BLEEDING

As an emergency measure, 4 grams Vitamin C taken all at once act as a haemostatic and will usually reduce the bleeding within an hour. See a doctor or other health professional as soon as possible to establish the cause of the bleeding.

Essential oil of Cypress reduces heavy bleeding in many instances but will have little effect if the bleeding is caused by fibroids, for example. Rub 3 drops, undiluted, into your belly. If the problem is long-term, use Cypress (6 drops) in your bath regularly. Be sure not to make the bath too hot.

Some women have found Iron phosphate helpful in the long term.

The herb Beth Root (Trillium erectum) is a valuable help: make a "tea" by simmering 1–2 teaspoons of dried herb to each cup of water and sipping one cupful three times a day. Or take 20 drops of beth Root tincture in a wineglassful of warm water three times a day. You can add a little honey to either the tea or the tincture if you like.

Always seek professional help, but keep up your self-help as well.

HOT FLUSHES

Camomile and Bergamot essential oils have a cooling effect. Use them in a cool bath (3 drops of each or 6 drops of either one).

Bergamot is an ingredient of classic eau de cologne which has a cooling effect if you use it as a body splash. Bergamot is the flavouring ingredient in Earl Grey tea and some women have found this helps – don't drink the tea too hot, though.

Fill a small spray bottle with rosewater and spray your face with it as needed.

Avoid clothes made of synthetic fibres. Choose cotton whenever possible and dress in several thin layers so that you can take the top layer off easily whenever you need to. In summer, wear skirts rather than trousers (and one lady of 70-plus advises wearing no knickers under your skirt).

The herb Agnus castus is very effective for preventing or reducing hot flushes and preparations based on it are available in most health-food shops. It appears to work best when used together with False Unicorn root: this combination is said to "remove 80 % of symptoms for 80% of women". If possible consult a medical herbalist who will work out the best combination for your personal needs.

Use all the methods suggested in this book for maintaining your hormone levels naturally.

Homoeopathy can be extremely helpful, but self-dosing is not advisable. Consult a properly trained homoeopath for an individually prescribed remedy.

If embarrassment is a big problem, try to remember that your hot flush is far less apparent to other people than it is to you.

CAUTION: Undiluted Bergamot on the skin can cause dangerous burning in sunny weather. Dilute before use, or restrict use to areas that won't be exposed to the sun, or stick to Camomile alone in summer.

LEAKING OF URINE

This can happen to even very young women after childbirth, especially when coughing, sneezing, taking exercise or lifting heavy weights.

Use the exercises described for prolapse in Chapter 17 (which were, in fact, developed by Kegel as a treatment for urinary problems and only later applied to prolapse.)

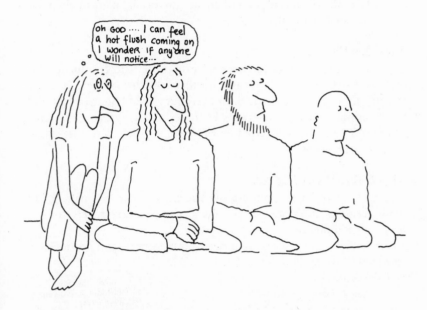

NIGHT SWEATS

Use any of the suggestions given above for hot flushes, plus:

A cool drink of Camomile tea before going to bed.

Use only cotton nighties, never synthetic. Avoid pyjamas.

Use cotton sheets rather than polyester or nylon mixtures. Avoid duvets with synthetic fillings. In fact, some say avoid duvets altogether and use light, cellular blankets.

Lay a bath towel over the bottom sheet with a small sheet over it (or use the best bits cut out of old sheets). This will save you having to change the whole bottom sheet if you do sweat.

Some women have found that two or three drops of Clary Sage essential oil massaged into the tummy before going to sleep helps to prevent sweats, but don't use Clary Sage if you have had any alcohol in the last few hours.

OSTEOPOROSIS

As preventive measures take regular exercise and make sure that your diet includes adequate calcium. See "Fuel for Life" and "Use It or Lose It" for details.

Use all the means described in this book to maintain your oestrogen levels naturally.

PROLAPSE

Use Kegel (pelvic floor) exercises for prevention and treatment, also exercise to strengthen thigh and buttock muscles as these increase the effectiveness of the pelvic floor exercises. (See "Use It or Lose It" for description of the exercises.) Exercises to strengthen abdominal ("tummy") muscles. Inverted yoga postures, but don't try these without supervision.

SEXUAL PROBLEMS

Talk to your partner: changing the pattern of your lovemaking can often get rid of problems due to menopausal changes, hysterectomy... or just plain boredom.

Difficulty with sex is often due to other stresses in a relationship. Specialised counselling usually helps enormously.

Essential oils of Clary Sage, Jasmine, Rose, Sandalwood, Ylang Ylang and several others are aphrodisiacs and can often help couples through a "bad patch". Use as a perfume, to massage each other, a drop on the pillow or a few drops in the bath before going to bed.

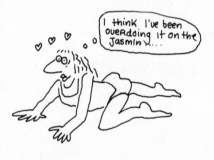

The herb Damiana may help, as may Ginseng. If you feel tense and stressed about your sexual relationship, try Lime Blossom tea, also the essential oil Neroli (Orange Blossom): both help to reduce tension surrounding sexual encounters.

Use pelvic muscle exercises to improve circulation in and around the sexual organs. Also, read the following entry.

VAGINAL DRYNESS.

In the short-term, use simple lubricants, such as water-based gels or pessaries, vegetable oil, unperfumed moisturisers or saliva (but no oil or oil-based creams or moisturisers at the same time as condoms.)

You can make your own "oestrogen" cream with essential oils of Clary Sage and Geranium and any pure, non-perfumed cream.

You'll find a formula in Appendix A.

Use oestrogen-like herbs such as Fennel, Hops or Liquorice to maintain your own hormone levels as much as possible.

Make sure your diet includes plenty of the foods and vitamins which help you to continue making oestrogen. See "Fuel for Life" for details.

Talk to your partner: slower foreplay is often all that is needed.

FURTHER READING:

Aromatherapy, An A-Z	Patricia Davis	*C.W. Daniel*
Bach Flower Remedies for Women	Judy Howard	*C.W. Daniel*
Dictionary of the Bach Flower Remedies	Hyne-Jones	*C.W. Daniel*
The New Holistic Herbal	D. Hoffmann	*Element*
Natural Healing in Gyneacology	R. Nissim	*Pandora*
A Woman's Herbal	Kitty Campion	*Arrow*

11

HRT – YES OR NO?

ONE OF THE biggest areas of controversy about menopause is the question of Hormone Replacement Therapy (HRT). Hormone Replacement Therapy has been hailed as a panacea, a recipe for eternal youth and the best thing that has happened to women this century. Famous women from pop stars to prime ministers have publicly proclaimed how wonderful it makes them feel. Others warn about its dangers and disadvantages just as vociferously. The truth, as with most things, lies somewhere between the extremes: there are some real benefits and there are some real dangers. Only you can decide whether, for you, the benefits outweigh the dangers or vice versa, and you can only make an informed choice when the facts are separated from the hype. So, let's have a look at what HRT is and what it can and cannot do.

One way of dealing with complications that may arise as oestrogen levels decline is to replace the "missing" hormones artificially. Tablets containing oestrogen or a mixture of oestrogen and progesterone are taken for three weeks each month and discontinued for a week, in the same manner as the contraceptive pill (though HRT does NOT give contraceptive protection). During the "off" week bleeding – an artificial period – is experienced, though very recent developments include formulations that avoid this. Hormones may also be prescribed in the form of an implant (a pellet inserted under the skin, which needs renewing every six months) or as skin patches like a sticking plaster, which need replacing every few weeks. A cream containing oestrogen is sometimes used locally if the main problem is vaginal dryness.

Oestrogen was first isolated (from sow's urine) in the 1930's but was not produced in commercially-useful quantities until the 1960's and has been used as a medical treatment for menopausal and post-menopausal problems since then. The hormones used may

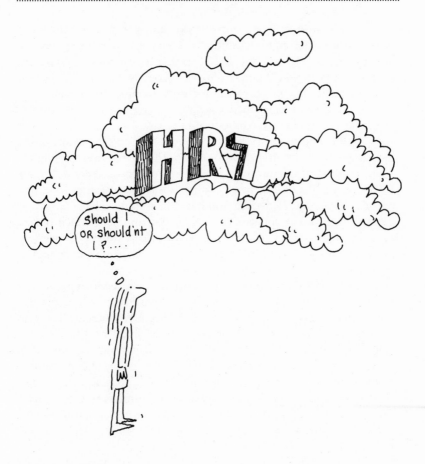

either be extracted from the urine of pregnant mares (equine hormones) or chemically manufactured. Some of the man-made hormones are described as synthetic, while others (which are nearer in their chemical structure to human hormones) are misleadingly called "natural" hormones. The synthetics are the least well tolerated by the body, and are less used than the other types.

The first replacement hormones were oestrogen only, but by the mid-70's it became clear that there was a connection between oestrogen replacement and certain cancers, but that if progesterone was also given, this risk was reduced. Progesterone is now usually given for 10 days in each cycle. This mimics the menstrual cycle more closely: during the first part of the cycle oestrogen prepares the lining of the womb (the endometrium) to receive a fertilised egg and the lining thickens. If no egg is fertilised, progesterone reverses the process and a period follows. When oestrogens were given alone as a replacement therapy, the endometrium became abnormally thick and some women developed cancers as a result. The addition of progesterone appears to have reduced this risk.

HRT effectively stops the hot flushes, night sweats, heavy bleeding and vaginal dryness associated with lowered oestrogen levels. More importantly, it protects against osteoporosis. Whether or not HRT reduces the risk of heart disease is less clear: studies have produced conflicting evidence. Some women using HRT report an improvement in the appearance of their skin and hair, which has led to this therapy being hailed as a recipe for eternal youth. (Conversely, it has led some doctors to regard it as a cosmetic measure and to treat women requesting HRT as frivolous.)

What HRT does not do (contrary to some media reports) is to help depression in most cases, or restore sexual drive where that has diminished. When a group of women taking HRT were studied only a tiny minority reported any improvement in libido or their ability to reach orgasm (though some women will feel sexier because their other discomforts have been relieved). Similarly, only about a third of women taking replacement hormones found that it helped their depression, and most doctors agree that hormone replacement is not the most appropriate help if a women's main problems are depression, anxiety or lethargy. In the same study, HRT was not found to have any beneficial effect on hair or skin.

Some women cannot take HRT at all for medical reasons. These include anybody who has had breast cancer, cancer of the endometrium or some other abnormalities of the endometrium.

You should not take replacement hormones if you suffer from endometriosis or fibroids, as it has been shown to make these conditions worse. If you have had a heart attack or stroke, thrombosis (blot-clots), hepatitis or other serious liver disorder HRT is not suitable for you and it may also be advised against if you are very overweight, have high blood pressure, smoke heavily or if there is a history of breast cancer in your family. If you have previously suffered from PMT, hormone replacement therapy can make this worse, and some women who have never previously suffered from this problem developed symptoms when taking HRT.

Your doctor should be able to advise you on all these points if you are considering whether or not HRT is the right solution for you. Unfortunately, I have heard of doctors prescribing this form of treatment after only minimal consultation, so it is as well to be aware of all the facts and ask as many questions as you need before making any decision. If you are not satisfied with the answers, ask to be referred to an endocrinologist. You have a right to a second opinion.

Some women decide not to use HRT because they dislike the idea of taking any drug on a long-term basis or because the treatment is still relatively new and its long-term side effects are far from fully documented. Vegans and many others will want to avoid using products derived from horses. Many women dislike the idea of indefinitely prolonging monthly bleeding: as one of them put it "I have this nightmare vision of tottering down to the chemist's on my zimmer-frame to pick up some tampons!" HRT does have to be used long-term because oestrogen levels drop again as soon as it is discontinued. Some doctors think it should be taken indefinitely, others reckon that ten years from the end of normal menstruation is long enough, especially if the therapy is being used to prevent osteoporosis, as this should delay the loss of calcium from the bones long enough to prevent abnormal fractures.

Some women who have tried HRT have discontinued it because they experienced nausea, breast tenderness, fluid retention, dizziness or other side-effects. Some have found that they felt abnormally nervous or highly-strung on this therapy. When I was discussing HRT with a reflexologist, she commented on some clients who were using replacement hormones "They're all like chestnut fillies!", accompanying her remark with a nervous twitch and toss of her head – and up to then she had not known that the hormones they were taking had probably been obtained from mares' urine!

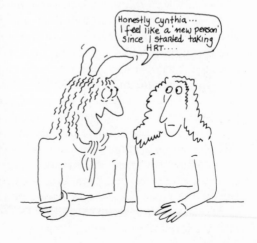

A fairly new concern about replacement hormones is that there is evidence to suggest that women can become addicted to them. Some women are needing higher doses to get the same effect or returning to their doctor or clinic for repeat treatment at shorter and shorter intervals, which suggests dependence.

The most serious concern about using replacement hormones, though, is that they do seem to increase the risk of certain cancers, especially breast cancer and some forms of cancer of the uterus. Women who are using HRT must be screened for these at much more frequent intervals than those who are not.

ALTERNATIVES TO HRT

If you need to make a decision whether or not to use HRT it may be useful to have an idea of some of the other options available.

If you want to stay within the area of orthodox medicine, there are alternatives to oestrogen or oestrogen/progesterone compounds. A progesterone-only prescription has been very successful in reducing or eliminating hot flushes. The drug Etidronate is being used successfully to prevent the development of osteoporosis. Vaginal dryness can be treated easily by applying an oestrogen cream locally: some oestrogen will be absorbed into the bloodstream but far less than with HRT. Creams containing testosterone (a male hormone) have been found effective, and are considered safe for women who cannot risk absorbing any oestrogen at all, for example, women who have had breast cancer. Alternatively, simple lubricating creams or gels are effective for women who do not want to use any kind of synthetic hormone.

If you want to avoid taking any form of drug, all of the alternative/complementary therapies described in Chapter 9 offer effective ways of reducing hot flushes, night sweats, vaginal dryness and other menopausal miseries.

Counselling or psychotherapy are safe and effective ways of handling depression, anxiety and sexual problems: safe because they do not rely on addictive tranquillisers, antidepressants, hormones or any other drug and effective because they help you to deal with the underlying causes rather than suppressing symptoms.

When we come to consider the two most serious conse-quences of lowered oestrogen levels – osteoporosis and the increased risk of heart disease – the orthodox and alternative views are the same, namely that relatively simple lifestyle changes are the most effective form of prevention.

You might also want to consider combining more than one approach. Even those who advocate HRT strongly agree that lifestyle improvements are important and it has been found that women who eat wisely and take some exercise can take much smaller doses of hormones.

Margot is a teacher with a long commitment to using natural therapies whenever possible. She exercises four or five times a week and her diet is very good. However, she is in a "high-risk" category for osteoporosis: she is petite, small-boned and comes from a family with a history of fractures among the older women. After a lot of thought she decided to take the minimum possible dosage of HRT and back this up with medicinal herbs. She is happy with this decision and feels that she is getting the best of both worlds.

Anna is a musician who had a total hysterectomy at the age of 35 (i.e., her ovaries were removed as well as her womb, producing an artificial menopause). This loss of natural oestrogen at a very early age puts her, too, at high risk of osteoporosis, although in her case there is no history of it among the older women in her family. Anna took HRT until she was 47 and then discontinued it, using a number of non-drug options instead. She combines herbal remedies, vitamin and mineral supplements, a good basic diet and regular exercise to keep her body healthy and her bones strong.

Such decisions are intensely personal: nobody else can make them for you and if anybody – doctor or otherwise – tries to pressurise you one way or another, ask for a second opinion and time to think about it while you weigh up all the pros and cons. As a long-time practitioner and user of alternative therapies I cannot hide my preference for non-drug based methods of maintaining health, but if I had been confronted with evidence that my bones were crumbling in my 40's or 50's I might have felt very differently.

12

TEN GOOD REASONS
FOR GIVING UP
SMOKING

DO YOU SMOKE? If you don't, you can skip this chapter, but if you do, PLEASE read on.

Yes, you've heard it all before, but I am going to say it all again because smoking is SO damaging to women at any age, and even more so as we get older, that if there was only one thing you could do to improve your health and well-being, giving up smoking would have to be it.

Smoking increases the risk of heart disease.

Smoking increases the risk of bronchitis and all lung diseases.

Smoking increases the risk of ALL cancers (not just lung cancer).

Smoking lowers the age at which you reach menopause (which increases other health risks).

Smoking destroys Vitamin C. in your body.

Smoking makes menopausal problems worse.

Smoking coarsens your skin.

Smoking encourages wrinkles.

Smoking makes you smell awful.

Smoking costs an awful lot of money.

If you have tried to give up smoking without success, get some help in giving it up now. If the biggest problem for you is physical craving, you might try nicotine lozenges or skin-patches which enable you to gradually decrease the amount of nicotine your body is getting over a period of three months or so. You can now buy these without prescription. If you find it impossible to stop smoking because of tension, anxiety or underlying emotional reasons you might ask your doctor to help, or look for an addiction counsellor or a self-help group to support you through the difficult period of weaning yourself off nicotine.

Don't tell yourself that you have smoked so long that giving up now is not going to make much difference to your health. The

GOOD news is that almost all the harmful effects of smoking can be reversed when you stop doing it, though obviously the sooner you stop, the more you will benefit.

FURTHER READING:

The Easy Way to Stop Smoking	Alan Carr	*Penguin*

13

KEEPING THE GREY CELLS ACTIVE

WHEN I TALK to other women about old age – and I mean 80, 90 and beyond – I realise that a common fear is of "going ga-ga". This fear is not exclusive to women of course: men and women alike have anxieties about losing their memory, becoming less capable intellectually, of "losing their marbles".

Why do some people lose much of their mental capacity as they age, while others have razor-sharp minds right to the end of their life? Even if we set aside considerations of illnesses that affect the mind, such as Alzheimer's Disease, we don't know all the answers to this question, but from what we do know it is clear that the maxim "use it or lose it" applies to your brain, just as much as to any other part of your body. The more work you give it to do, the more efficiently it will work. Studies of older people have shown that even something as simple as doing crossword puzzles helps prevent memory loss.

You might not enjoy solving crossword puzzles, but they are a good illustration of what is needed to keep the brain active, and active is the operative word: the difference between doing the crossword and simply reading the newspaper or magazine in which it appears is that you have to DO something in response to what you are reading. You have to interact with the printed page.

But that's not quite the whole story. Crosswords specifically exercise the part of the brain that deals with words, the logical, verbal part of the brain: the left hemisphere. Solving mathematical problems, playing chess, doing anything that involves logic and reasoning engages the left hemisphere, too.

Different parts of the brain are associated with different kinds of thinking and, loosely speaking, the left brain (or hemisphere) deals with logic, reasoning, organization while the right brain is more involved with intuition, creativity and non-verbal expression.

Of course, this is an over-simplification, and almost anything that you do in life involves all parts of the brain. A musician, for example, may work very much from the right brain in terms of inspiration or original melodies, but it takes plenty of left-brain input to organise that first inspiration into a composition and get it all down on paper. Conversely, we tend to think of science as a logical, left-brain activity but virtually every great scientific discovery has originated with a sudden flash of insight. It may have taken years of logical, theoretical work thereafter to establish the truth of that first idea, but without the intuitive, right-brain, flash there would not have been a theory in the first place.

So, if you want your brain to be active when you are 90, give it plenty of work to do now! And, if possible, give it a variety of challenges so that you exercise all of it. If you are logical and intellectual by inclination, it would be good to engage in some creative activity sometimes: join a dance class, paint or sing in a choir. If you are more intuitive by nature and inclined towards non-verbal, artistic activities, try learning chess, or buy a book of logic puzzles or......do the crossword!

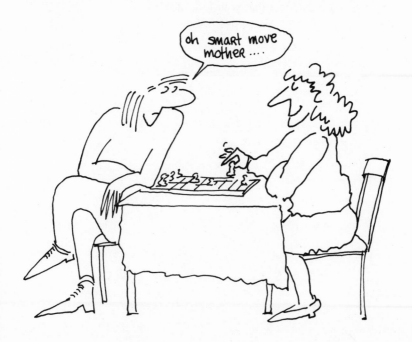

A lot of women in mid-life say that they lack mental stimulus. This may be because they have spent 20 to 30 years keeping house and child rearing and feel that this does not challenge them enough intellectually, or it may be that they have been doing a job outside the home that has become repetitive and unsatisfying. Even women who have been doing both at once often fail to get a lot of mental satisfaction from this mammoth juggling act and say that they are too exhausted at the end of the day to do anything that requires mental effort.

Ironically, doing something a little bit challenging and outside of their normal routine, however tiring that may be, would probably help them to feel less exhausted. The feeling of tiredness often arises from the repetitive nature of their everyday work and the fact that they don't have to make much mental effort to carry them out. Engaging the brain in something new, especially if it is quite different from the daily round, is a really good antidote. And, most important of all, it helps to ensure that the mind stays alert and effective for decades to come.

So don't just sit there – DO SOMETHING! What you do doesn't matter: the fact that you do it, does.

14

LOOKING AFTER YOUR APPEARANCE

M ANY WOMEN ARE anxious about the way their appearance may change as they pass through menopause. Sometimes these fears mask deeper ones: worrying about wrinkles or grey hair may stem from fears about other aspects of growing older. I have seen this repeatedly in my aromatherapy practice: a new client books in for facial massage, she is bothered about the wrinkles around her eyes or saggy skin on her neck but after perhaps two or three treatments she begins to confide her real concerns. There is often fear of becoming less sexually desirable, perhaps of losing a partner because of this or it may be that these first wrinkles have brought up issues around old age, sickness and death. But much needless misery is caused by media images and social attitudes that equate beauty with youth. We have few examples of beautiful older women as role models. Film actresses who are described as "still beautiful" in their 50's are nearly always those who strive to preserve an illusion of youth via facelifts, breast lifts, bum lifts, hair dyes and anorexic diets.

So before we go any further, I want to assert that YOU CAN BE BEAUTIFUL AT ANY AGE.

You do not have to be an imitation teenager to be attractive.

Every age has its own beauty, and a woman of 80 who wears her wrinkles gracefully can be far more charming than the woman of 40 who tries to hide them.

This doesn't mean, though, that we should not maximise our looks and enjoy doing so. Choosing clothes, cosmetics and hairstyles is FUN. But we need to start from inside, because the appearance of our skin, hair and nails depends on their health and that relates very much to our general health. If you make sure that you have good nutrition, appropriate exercise and enough sleep, your appearance should be pretty good. It will certainly be better than that of women who eat junk and don't exercise. Once you have established this firm base, there are a few things you should know about skincare, etc., that will help you look your very best.

The first thing to understand is that changes in your appearance, especially your skin, have very little to do with menopause but are part of the general process of aging. This is illustrated by the fact that women who have a very early menopause, or young women who have had their ovaries removed for medical reasons producing an artificial menopause, do not develop wrinkles any earlier than those who reach menopause late.

The only connection between skin aging and menopause is that oestrogen helps to maintain the elasticity of collagen. Collagen forms much of the underlying layer of our skin, and helps to make it firm and smooth. But other factors affect collagen, too, especially nutrition, so a post-menopausal woman who eats wisely may have a smoother and firmer skin than a young woman who doesn't.

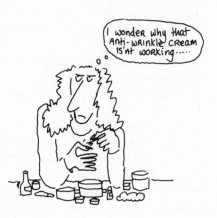

Androgens – the "male" hormones which women produce throughout life in their ovaries and adrenal glands – also help to keep the skin firm, so everything that affects the health of your ovaries and adrenals affects your skin, too.

TAKING CARE OF YOUR SKIN

Choosing the right skincare products is more important in mid-life and after than in your teens. This doesn't mean spending a fortune on anti-wrinkle creams or hyped-up "cell regenerators".The best products for older skins are often simple ones and don't have to be expensive. Look for ranges based on plant oils and extracts rather than mineral oils, animal fats and man-made chemicals. Plants oils and extracts provide us with elements that our skin needs in a form that it can easily absorb. Mineral oils, on the other hand, are not easily absorbed but "sit" on the surface of the skin. Animal fats, such as lanolin, are often used as a base for creams but some people are allergic to lanolin and others do not wish to use animal fats for ethical reasons. If you want to avoid them, there are plenty of products which contain no animal materials and are not tested on animals: this will always be stated on the labels.

Learn to read the labels as critically as you would when buying food: some items with "natural" sounding names have only a tiny amount of a plant extract in an otherwise mineral/chemical mixture. Look for products that state clearly that they contain ONLY plant materials, or which list their ingredients. You are more likely to find such products in health-food stores than cosmetic departments.

Use unperfumed products, or those that contain natural perfumes only (essential oils or plant extracts). Synthetic perfumes can produce allergic reactions and, at best, they do nothing. Essential oils, on the other hand, do far more than perfume your cream or lotion. They have many beneficial actions, depending on which oil, or combination of oils, is used. Some essential oils which are particularly beneficial for older skins are Rose, Jasmine, Sandalwood and Frankincense. Rose is especially good if your skin is dry and sensitive, while Frankincense is one of the few substances in nature that really does have an effect on wrinkles!

Using Frankincense regularly on the skin helps to prevent wrinkles forming, and it can even iron out existing ones to a certain extent though it takes time and really regular use to do so.

Avoid toners with a lot of alcohol in them: they strip the natural oils from the skin. Young skins are rich in sebum (natural oil) and can withstand alcohol-based toners or astringents, but from our mid-thirties onwards we secrete less sebum and need to conserve what we have, as it protects the skin from atmospheric pollution, bacteria and the drying effects of wind outdoors and central heating indoors. Your toner should only remove your cleanser, not this protective layer. Simple rosewater will do this perfectly well.

If possible, treat yourself to the luxury of a facial massage by a trained aromatherapist who will be able to suggest the most appropriate oils for your skin. Failing that, or between treatments, you could make your own massage oil by adding a few drops of essential oil to a good quality vegetable oil. Put 2 drops of Rose oil (or Jasmine, Sandalwood, etc.) in 5 mls. of avocado or peach kernel oil for a luxurious face treatment. Massage this gently into your face and leave it on for at least 20 minutes and clean off any surplus gently with rosewater.

You can also add any of these oils to unperfumed creams if

you prefer: stir 12 drops of essential oil to each ounce (30 gms) of cream. If you like, you can blend two or more essential oils together, so long as you don't exceed the total of 12 drops to each ounce of base cream.

A WORD ABOUT WEIGHT

Just about the worst thing you can do in mid-life is go on a crash diet! Drastic weight-loss has many negative implications for your health, and as far as appearance is concerned, you're likely to end up looking haggard and ill. Although we know that a slight reduction in calorie intake, and therefore in weight, helps to slow down the aging process, it is essential that this is done gradually. If you do need to lose weight, don't reduce your calorie intake too much. Some women will lose weight easily on 1,500 cals while others might need to go as low as 1,200. Less than 1,000 is really dangerous: you are likely to lose lean muscle and – even more dangerous – bone mass.

On such a regime, you can expect to drop about 3 lbs in the first week and 1 lb a week after that. That's a safe and healthy rate and it doesn't matter if it takes several months, or even a year, to reach your ideal weight. Two or three exercise sessions a week will help you tone up muscles. Dropping weight by eating less alone – without exercise – can leave you very flabby.

But do you really need to lose weight? Are you being realistic about it? Of course, obesity is dangerous, but if you weigh 7 or 8 lbs more than when you were 25 that is perfectly alright. Remember that androgens are converted into oestrogens in your fat cells, so a few more fat cells actually make for a smoother passage through menopause. Middle-aged spread is one of nature's ways of helping us maintain our oestrogen levels.

15

MAKING FRIENDS WITH YOUR BODY

HOW WELL DO you know your own body? And how much do you like it?

I don't think I have ever met a woman who liked every aspect of her own body: even beautiful women who most of us would think of as "perfect" and perhaps envy for that.

Dislike for one's own body can become acute in middle age if we begin to compare ourselves unfavourably with younger women, or with the image of ourselves ten or twenty years ago. But a negative self-image is very destructive, and if you want your body to carry you on into a vigorous and healthy old age, it's a good idea to start thinking of it as a friend.

Here's an exercise for you to try: get a pencil and paper and write down ten things you like about your body. Do this as quickly as you can: don't think about it too much. If you can't find ten items easily, stop. If you have got to ten and can still think of a lot more, keep on writing. When you've finished, draw a line and do the same again but listing the things you don't like about your body. Now compare the two lists. Which was the longest? Were all the items you listed externals, such as blue eyes, nice hair or did you include such things as strong muscles, a good digestion or other less visible assets? Did you find it difficult to do this exercise? How easy was it to find ten things you really like about your body? There aren't any "right" or "wrong" answers to this exercise, it is just one way of finding out how you feel about your body.

If you found it hard to identify ten things you like about your body it is worth exploring ways of improving your self-image. There are many ways you might go about this. For example, you might make a list of everything you like about yourself that has nothing to do with your body. You might ask your friends to write down the ten things they like most about you (ask your friends to be honest and explain that you are not fishing for compliments!). You may well find that not one item relates to your body and that what your friends value are qualities such as compassion, humour, honesty or sensitivity

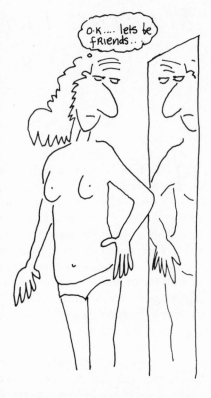

Natasha, who felt very negative about her body, which she saw as "fat" was amazed to discover that none of her friends thought of her as overweight – they just saw the lovely and loving person that she was. For much of her life she had held the belief "Nobody loves me" and comforted herself with food, even though she knew this made her fatter, until the belief became "Nobody loves me because I'm fat". The realization that she was, indeed, very much loved and that the shape and size of her body had nothing to do with this, was a turning point for Natasha. Separating her appearance from her feelings about love was the first step towards loving herself more.

Often, we project onto our physical appearance some aspect of our personality or behaviour that we feel bad about, so "I don't like my saggy tummy" may be covering up a more hurtful truth such as "I don't like myself because I'm lazy and don't take enough exercise." Because of this, starting an exercise programme (or anything else that might help) can increase our positive feelings about ourselves out of all proportion to any physical effect.

At mid-life, we may also project outwards our fears about growing older and the changes that have taken place, or are taking place, in our bodies. Go back to your list of "Don't likes" and put a cross against anything that relates specifically to growing older, such as "wrinkles" or "greying hair". Just sit quietly for a few minutes and ask yourself why you dislike these aspects of your appearance: do they trigger hidden anxieties? are you afraid of getting older? are you comparing yourself unfavourably with younger women? or with yourself when you were young? Are you afraid that your mature body will be less attractive to your partner?

All these issues confront us at menopause, and they need to be dealt with. Talking about them honestly with other women often helps, either one-to-one with a friend, or in a women's group, or maybe in counselling or therapy. But don't confuse them with the way you see your body.

Making friends with your body goes much further than learning to like it. It also means treating it kindly, finding out what are its real needs, and – as far as possible – meeting those needs.

However you feel about your body, it is your oldest and closest companion. It's been with you from the beginning of your life and it will be with you to the end. Even if you have suffered much illness and pain, or permanent disability, your body is the vehicle in which you are living this human life and if you think of menopause as a halfway point in your journey through life, it is a good moment to stop and consider how well you are treating the vehicle.

It's a time to start listening to your body: finding out what its real needs are. For example, how much sleep does it need? Which foods make it feel good? Or bad?

By "listening" I mean taking a few moments each day to notice how you are feeling physically. It is very easy to ignore the state of your own body if you lead a busy life: so many of us have learnt to override fatigue, minor illness and pain to meet work deadlines or the needs of other people. Women and girls are often conditioned from a very young age to be aware of other people's needs: "Ssh, Daddy's got a headache" slips almost unnoticed into "Ssh, the boss has got a headache". Mothers, especially, learn to be ultra-sensitive to their children's physical needs. They know what foods upset this one's tummy, what time that one needs to go to bed, when to call the doctor and how much excitement is too much.

How many of us understand our own bodies so well? Very few, I suspect.

It's really just a question of being aware: in the mornings, notice whether you feel better after 8 hours sleep, or 6 hours, or less, or more. If you feel sluggish or bloated after a meal, remember what you ate. Next time you have a headache, think back a few hours and see if you can work out whether a stuffy room, a long drive, a heavy lunch or maybe eyestrain might be the cause. When you are feeling stressed, ask yourself how long it is since you allowed yourself time to do something just for you, something you really enjoy.

Of course, once you have identified what makes you feel good and what makes you feel bad, you need to DO something about it! Go to bed earlier, or get up earlier, or cut cheese out of your diet for a week or two, or lie in a perfumed bath for two hours with a book: whatever makes you feel great.

It isn't only your body that deserves such care. You need to look after your other needs, too. Does your work satisfy you – whether it is computer programming or feeding a family? Are you nourished by the music you hear, the TV you watch, the books you read? Do you spend enough time with your friends? Or, conversely, do you allow yourself enough time to be alone quietly, if that is what you need? If you have a creative activity, do you have enough time to practise it?

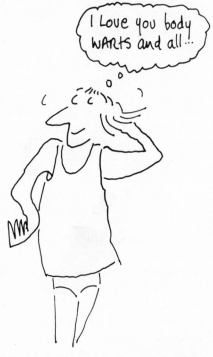

Learning to love yourself and look after yourself in all these ways isn't always easy. Even if you can overcome old habits of putting work, partner or family before your own needs, you may meet resistance from the people around you especially if they are used to you behaving like a doormat. If you feel guilty about spending even a few minutes on yourself, consider how much better a cared-for body will serve you in every area of your life. Tell yourself (and anybody else who needs to hear this) that your body has served you well for forty or fifty years and that you intend to take care of it so that it will continue to serve you well for many years to come.

Cherish yourself. You deserve it.

16

FUEL FOR LIFE

WHAT WE EAT really does make a difference to our health and as we grow older, this becomes more apparent. Young people can eat junk foods and wash them down with sugar-rich fizzy drinks and show no ill effects, beyond the odd pimple or two, for many years. The effects of poor diet in youth may not become apparent until mid-life or later and while we cannot always undo completely the effect of earlier bad habits, we can improve our health at any age by giving some thought to what we put into our bodies.

Food provides us with the "building-blocks" of life, the materials that we need to make new cells. Some of the cells that make up all the different organs and tissues of our bodies are dying all the time and new ones forming. As we grow older, forming new cells to repair and maintain body tissues becomes an important consideration but our bodies may have got less efficient at extracting all the necessary nutrients from our food, so it helps to choose foods carefully to provide the body with all the elements that it needs.

By giving some care to what we eat and how we prepare it, we can reduce the risk of certain illnesses and, to some extent, slow down the process of aging. This doesn't mean trying to live for ever – it means giving yourself the best chances of leading a healthy, active and enjoyable life for many years ahead.

Food For Strong Bones
To maintain the strength of your bones you need calcium. I'm sure you know already that milk and cheese are a prime source of calcium and for many people they are a good choice and easy to obtain. The disadvantage is that they are high in animal fats which contribute to heart disease, so if milk is going to be your main source of calcium, use the skimmed kind - it has just as much as whole milk. Skimmed milk powder is very rich in calcium, so you could add a spoonful to

cereals and cooked dishes. Yoghurt is comparable to milk in calcium content and is more easily digested but, here again, choose the low-fat varieties. If you make your own yoghurt, add some skimmed milk powder to the milk at the beginning to increase the calcium content. Goat's milk is a fraction higher in calcium than cow's milk, and ewe's milk is much higher, so yoghurts and cheeses made from them are an excellent source.

Hard cheeses provide more calcium than soft ones, with Parmesan, Emmenthal, Gruyere, Gouda, Cheddar and Edam giving good amounts (in that order). Unfortunately, most hard cheeses are higher in saturated fats than soft ones so limit your intake, especially if you are post-menopausal when you run more risk of heart disease.

Vegans will not use dairy produce (or any other product derived from animals) for ethical reasons, and an increasing number of people are avoiding dairy produce because of food allergies or sensitivities. If you don't take milk, you will have to work a bit harder at getting your calcium, but there are many good sources from nuts, seeds, vegetables and legumes.

Make friends with the soya bean and its derivatives. Tofu (soya bean curd) contains more calcium than any non-animal food except sesame seeds. It is difficult to eat sesame seeds in sufficient quantities to meet your calcium needs but tahini (sesame seed paste) provides the same amount in a more convenient form. Soya milk is much lower in calcium than cows' milk, although some brands have calcium added – read the labels.

The following vegetable foods are listed in order of their calcium content – the highest first: sesame seeds and tahini, tofu, sunflower seeds, soya beans, almonds, kale, soya flour, dried figs, watercress, red kidney beans, pistachio nuts, brazil nuts, broccoli, mung beans and chick peas. Other nuts, legumes and dark green vegetables contain useful amounts, so try to include a wide variety of them in your diet even if you use dairy produce as well. There is good evidence that obtaining your calcium in several different forms increases absorption.

If you are happy to include fish in your diet, tinned salmon, pilchards and mackerel are a good source, provided you eat the tiny bones.

Getting enough calcium is not the whole story, though: you also need Vitamins A and D, magnesium and some other minerals to fix it in your bones and you need to avoid some foods and other substances that prevent fixing.

Without enough magnesium, calcium may be deposited in your joints instead of in the bones, giving you a lot of pain, or in soft tissues where it may be equally damaging. An ideal ratio is one part of magnesium to every two parts of calcium. The following foods are rich in both calcium and magnesium: broccoli, peas, peanut butter, tinned sardines, tinned salmon, tofu, brown rice, raisins and almonds.

The calcium in food doesn't all get into your bones. Some gets lost in the digestive process and certain foods, medicines and other substances increase the amount lost. To make sure your body really uses the calcium you eat, try to avoid the following "baddies":

Alcohol This prevents proper digestion of calcium. Alcoholics may lose as much bone mass by the age of 45 as non-alcoholics lose by 65. One glass of wine a day (preferably organic) is the safe limit.

Aluminium salts Some antacids prescribed for indigestion contain aluminium salts, which dissolve calcium. If you get antacids on prescription ask your doctor about this. If you buy them over the counter, read the labels or ask the pharmacist. Avoid cooking in aluminium saucepans, etc. Apart from calcium loss, there are other very good reasons for avoiding aluminium, not least because it is suspected of contributing to Alzheimer's disease.

Coffee There are substances in coffee, tea and chocolate which prevent calcium digestion, so try to limit these to two cups a day at the most. Most of the baddies are still present in decaffeinated versions and some brands use aluminium salts to remove the caffeine. If you want to drink decaffeinated tea or coffee, check with the manufacturer that it has been treated by the water process only.

Acids Acids dissolve calcium so that it flushes straight out in your urine. They include tannic acid in tea, oxalic acid in spinach and rhubarb and phytic acid in some grains. Phytic acid is concentrated in the outer husk (bran) and too great an intake of bran-based cereals has been shown to influence calcium absorption. It's safer to get your fibre from a variety of sources, such as fresh fruit, vegetables and whole grains rather than relying on bran alone to provide you with all the fibre you need.

Excess protein Most people in the West eat too much protein, sometimes twice as much as their bodies need. This interferes with calcium absorption, especially if the protein is mostly from red meats. The reasons are not yet fully understood, but seem to be related to the acid/alkaline balance of our systems. Our bodies work best when they are slightly alkaline and if the balance is too acidic, much of the calcium we get from food is used up simply neutralising the acids. Meat produces an acidic reaction in the body, and lacto-vegetarians (people who eat dairy produce as well as vegetable foods, but no meat) have been found to have a bone density in their seventies equal to that of meat-eaters in their fifties.

Phosphorous This is one of the components of bone, but too much of it prevents calcium fixing. Most people get too much phosphorus in their food because of the wide use of phosphates in agriculture and food processing. The amount of phosphates in meat is another possible reason why heavy meat eating prevents calcium absorption. If possible, buy organic vegetables, fruits, grains, etc. as no phosphates will have been used in growing them. In many places it is also possible to get meat from organically reared animals. Avoid processed foods as much as you can, also colas and other fizzy drinks as they are high in phosphorus.

Supplements Even with a good diet you may need to use supplements to get enough calcium, especially if you are menopausal, post-menopausal, pregnant or lactating. Women need 1,200–1,500 mgs daily after 35 and between 1,500–2,000 mgs daily by the age of 70. Most people get about 450 mgs a day from food, but this may be as little as 300 mgs if you don't eat dairy produce. To protect your bones you need to make up the difference with a supplement. Multimineral or vitamin/mineral supplements seldom contain enough calcium, for reasons of sheer size. Calcium is bulky and enough for one day usually has to be divided into three or four tablets. Divide them into three doses, two to be taken with meals and a larger amount to be taken at bedtime, because your body uses more calcium while you are asleep. It will help with insomnia, too. The traditional hot, milky drink at bedtime does the same thing.

Many calcium supplements also contain magnesium in the correct ratio, so check labels for this. If not, look for a supplement that will give you half as much magnesium as your daily intake of calcium (though it will almost certainly be cheaper to find a brand that combines both, as well as more convenient – less different pills to swallow).

Vitamin D, essential to bone health, is made in our bodies provided we get enough sunlight. 15 minutes a day out of doors is enough in the summer, but in winter you need an hour each day. If this is not possible you might like to add a supplement in winter only.

Vitamins C and E are needed for healthy collagen – the material that binds together all the minerals in your bones. We cannot make Vitamin C in our own bodies so we depend for it entirely on food sources. Fresh fruit and green vegetables are the main providers but it is a fragile vitamin and easily lost in cooking or storage. We also need a lot more when we are ill or stressed, so you may want to take a supplement at such times, even if you get plenty from natural sources, which is always the best way. Remember also that this vitamin cannot be stored in the body, so you need to get some from your food every day.

There is a tendency for collagen to weaken and lose its elasticity as we grow older, so women over 50 need to increase their intake of Vitamin C. Make sure you get 1,000 mgs (1 gram) a day regularly and up to 5 grams a day when you are stressed or unwell. There is absolutely no danger in taking large amounts of Vitamin C because it is a water-soluble vitamin, so if you take too much it just flushed out of your body. It is a good idea, though, to divide your daily requirements into three or four small doses so that your body uses it efficiently. A single large dose just produces rather expensive urine!

Vitamins C and E work best in combination with each other. To ensure that you really use all your Vitamin C, you need up to 400 I.U.s (International Units) a day of Vitamin E.

FOOD FOR A HEALTHY HEART

To maintain good cardiovascular health, we need to choose foods that benefit our veins and arteries, and avoid foods that damage them. You probably know quite a bit already about the foods to avoid, as this aspect of healthy eating is written and talked about much more than some other areas of nutrition, but it will do no harm to repeat here some of the major "no-no's".

Chief among these are saturated fats. Most saturated fats are animal fats, found in meat and dairy produce. A sensible approach is to choose lean meats, if you wish to eat meat at all, cut off all visible fat and use cooking methods that do not add more fat. Throw away the frying pan and use the grill instead. Baste with stock rather than fat when roasting, and skim all visible fat off the top of gravies, sauces, stocks, etc. (It helps to let them cool completely or even put them in the fridge, when the fat will solidify and is then much easier to remove.)

Red meats in general are heavier in fat than poultry but when eating chicken or turkey, remember that most of the fat is in and immediately below the skin, so avoiding the skin will reduce the amount of fat you are eating. If you are cooking chicken in a casserole, etc., remove the skin before cooking, otherwise remove it afterwards. Game meats such as venison are now quite widely available in butchers' shops and are also a healthier option than beef or pork.

Among dairy products, choose low-fat cheeses, skimmed or semi-skimmed milk and low-fat yoghurts which will give you just as much protein and calcium as the high-fat varieties. Remember that soft cheeses, in general, contain less fat than the hard ones.

Butter is a slightly controversial topic: it is concentrated animal fat and many people choose vegetable-oil margarines for that reason, but the processes used to solidify those vegetable oils may be as damaging as the animal fat because of the formation of free-radicals (which are discussed a bit further on). Current thinking is that a LITTLE butter is a safer choice than margarine. It's worth asking yourself whether you really need a fatty spread on your bread/toast/ crispbread if you are going to put jam, marmalade or a savoury spread on top. If you are making sandwiches to be eaten hours later, a thin spread of butter will stop the filling soaking into the bread, but for anything you are going to eat straight away, you might find you can perfectly well do without. This is also a very easy way to loose weight, if that is something you need to do. Butter and other fats are the most concentrated source of calories there is, and cutting down fat intake will cut down the fat on you, too!

You probably know already that alcohol contributes to high blood pressure and heart disease. This is because it reduces the elasticity of the artery walls. This does not mean that you have to cut out alcohol completely but it makes sense to avoid the spirits and keep other alcohol to a moderate level. There is some evidence to show that a LITTLE wine with meals is actually beneficial to the health of the heart.

Salt is the next thing you need to steer clear of as this, too contributes to high blood pressure, placing additional strain on the heart. We can get all the salt our bodies need from what is present naturally in foods – and I do mean naturally, not salt that has been added during processing and cooking. Try to stop adding salt altogether, your food need not taste insipid as a result. Steaming vegetables instead of boiling them retains all their flavour, so you won't need added seasoning. Herbs and spices can make dishes really interesting without added salt, or with very little. If you've been used to lots of salt in food and find it difficult to make such changes, there are salt substitutes and low-salt condiments in many shops. Watch out for the "hidden" salt in processed and ready-cooked foods. it turns up everywhere, even in sweet foods such as cakes, biscuits and deserts.

On the subject of sweet things sugar, of course, is another food to avoid, though sugar is not really a food at all as it does not provide us with a single thing that our bodies need. Nutritionists often refer to sugar as "empty calories" meaning that it adds a large number of calories to our daily intake without providing any nutrients. Because of that, it contributes to problems with weight and that in turn puts unnecessary stress on the heart. Sugar also destroys Vitamin C in the body, and C is one of the most important vitamins for the health of the blood-vessels.

You've already read about collagen in the chapter about your bones, but collagen is found throughout the body, binding other tissues together, strengthening them and keeping them elastic. The blood vessels are no exception: collagen keeps the walls of the arteries strong and pliable. You will remember that Vitamins C and E are essential to the elasticity of collagen and there is now good evidence that Vitamin C can even repair some of the damaged collagen when artery walls have begun to harden. These two vitamins work best together, so make sure you include foods that provide both. Plenty of fresh vegetables and fruit will supply Vitamin C and you can get Vitamin E from nuts and seeds, wheatgerm, milk, egg yolks, dark leaf vegetables such as spinach and broccoli and unrefined vegetable oils.

Supplements

If you feel you are not getting enough Vitamins C and E from food-stuffs, if you are ill or stressed, or if you already have high blood pressure, a heart disorder or circulatory problems such as varicose veins, it would be sensible to add them to your diet in the form of supplements. Check the entry above for suitable amounts. Garlic contains a variety of minerals and trace elements that contribute to cardiovascular health, so use it frequently in food if you enjoy the flavour. If not, take it daily in the form of odourless capsules.

ANTI-CANCER FOODS

The link between diet and cancer was first made when Western doctors noticed that cancer is very rare among people who have not adopted 20th century "civilisation" but preserved their traditional ways of living and eating. Their traditional diets vary according to the part of the world where they live and what is locally available. What is common to all of them, though, is that their food has not been through any form of processing (other than drying in some cases) no salt is added and in many places sugar is unknown and honey the only sweetener. These people tend to eat mainly grains and vegetables with a little fish or meat and fruits that are in season or which they can preserve themselves by drying. Grains and the flours made from them are not refined (in other words, the whole of the grain is used). Such a diet is very close to what our earliest ancestors ate.

The first observation that doctors made was that cancer of the intestines was virtually unknown and the crucial factor seemed to be that these unrefined foods pass through the intestines much faster than a typical Western diet. Foods that take a long time to move through the gut start to decompose before they are eliminated from the body and release all kinds of toxic by-products into the intestines. These get absorbed into the body along with, and sometimes instead of, the nutrients that we need.

The relationship between food and cancers of the intestines is a fairly direct one, but later observations showed that other cancers were also rare among people who ate in this way. Because these people mostly live in remote, unindustrialised areas it was thought that the absence of stress and pollution might be a major factor, rather than the type of diet, but when such people adopt a "Western" diet, they very quickly develop all the diseases that were previously rare among them. So it seems that although pollution is a factor affecting our health, what we eat is a more important one.

Apart from passing quickly through the digestive system, the other significant fact about a diet that does not include any processed foods is that it is free from any artificial additives: colourings, flavourings, preservatives, emulsifiers and so forth. We know now that many of these substances are carcinogens – they directly cause cancer. Even those that have been approved by various governments as "safe" are thought by many health professionals to be suspect.

Many of the pesticides and herbicides used in commercial fruit and vegetable production are suspect, too.

Other possible cancer-promoting substances in food are the hormones fed to poultry, beef and dairy cattle. We know that some cancers are hormone-linked, so it makes sense to avoid ingesting hormones in our food, particularly as we have no way of knowing what quantities may be involved.

A relatively recent discovery has been the role of free radicals. Free radicals are molecules that are short of one electron. Because molecules usually have their electrons in pairs, a free radical whizzes around among the molecules of your body trying to pull an extra electron out of an existing pair – rather like the vamp at a cocktail party! This leaves the other molecule short of an electron so it pulls one out of another pair.....and so on! A single free radical can generate thousands of others in this way. The danger of such a chain reaction in the body is that it damages the molecules that make up our body cells and can distort DNA, the genetic material which contains the "codes" that enable cells to reproduce themselves. If it is damaged the new cells may not be perfect copies of the ones they were meant to replace. Cancers may form when cells reproduce abnormaly.

Free radicals occur naturally in the body as a by-product of normal metabolism, but their levels are increased by many external factors, such as air pollution (especially car exhausts and waste products from industry), ultra-violet light, what we eat and how we cook it. The risk from ultra-violet light is increasing because of the thinning of the ozone layer. In the short term, you cannot change the environmental factors, but you CAN make decisions about what you eat and how you cook it. In the long term, of course, you can influence the ozone layer and the state of the air by your lifestyle choices and via environmental pressure groups.

As far as food is concerned, the levels are affected by the amount and type of fats we eat, and how we cook. Free radicals are formed when fats oxidise. This can happen slowly, when butter, margarine, oils, etc. are exposed to the air or it can happen quickly when they are heated. (The bad smell of rancid fats is a result of oxidisation.) Some of the processes used in turning vegetable oils into margarine produce free radicals, too, and many nutritionists feel that a LITTLE butter is a safer choice than margarine for that reason.

The heat used in the extraction of vegetable oils can also lead to free radical formation, so look for cold-pressed oils: olive, sunflower, etc. (If the label does not state that the oil is cold-pressed, it is almost certainly not.) Keep your good oils in the fridge, not on a shelf or in a cupboard.

Oxidization also takes place when you heat fats during cooking, especially at the high temperatures needed for frying. Some oils oxidize at much lower temperatures than others, so use a little olive oil if you really need to fry anything, as it can be heated to far higher temperatures than other oils before any changes take place. Avoid foods such as crisps and roasted peanuts which involve very hot fats in their preparation.

Fortunately, there are certain vitamins and minerals which inactivate free radicals. They do so by releasing one of their own electrons before decaying harmlessly. Vitamins A, C and E and the mineral selenium all have this action and are sometimes referred to as free-radical "scavengers". All four of them protect the body in other ways, too, such as strengthening the immune system so include plenty of them in your diet every day.

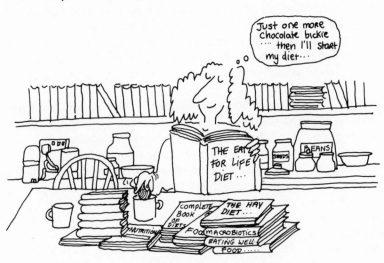

Vitamin C, as you almost certainly know, is found in most fresh fruits and vegetables. We can neither make nor store it in the body, so we need to take in enough each day from food or supplements. It is easily destroyed in cooking, so raw fruits, salads or very lightly steamed vegetables are the best source.

Vitamin A is made in the body from beta carotene, found in

green, orange and yellow fruits and vegetables, especially carrots, spinach and other green leaf vegetables, also in liver and some fish. It is stored in the liver, and too much of it over a long time can be dangerous, so it is better to get this from food sources rather than supplements. If you eat very little of the foods that provide Vitamin A or beta carotene, you may need a supplement but don't take more than the amount recommended by the manufacturer.

Vitamin E is found in vegetable oils, nuts, seeds, wholegrains, some fish and smaller amounts in fruits and vegetables. Although it is stored in the body like Vitamin A, quite large amounts can be tolerated without harm. Once again, use a supplement if your food is unlikely to give you enough.

Selenium is a mineral which our bodies need to make an enzyme that helps to prevent damage from free radicals. How much of this enzyme we can make depends, up to a point, on how much selenium we get.

Women with breast cancer and other cancer sufferers have been found to have very low levels of selenium in their blood stream.

Selenium occurs abundantly in the soil in some parts of the world but is scarce or absent in others. In places where deaths from cancer are above average, it has been found that there is very little selenium in the soil. It is found in liver, fish, lamb, prawns, milk, eggs also brown rice and some other grains but the amount varies a great deal according to where the food originated. Although there are some regional variations, soils in the U.K. are mostly deficient in selenium. From mid-life onwards, it is prudent to take it in the form of a supplement, particularly if you eat little or no meat or fish. 250 micrograms a day is a suitable amount for most women.

So what can we learn from all this that will help to protect us from cancer?

To eat plenty of foods that pass quickly through the gut. This means fresh vegetables and fruits, salads, beans, seeds, nuts, whole grains (wholewheat, brown rice, etc.) and wholegrain products (wholewheat bread, natural muesli, etc.)

To avoid foods that have a slow passage through the gut. This means fats, meat, sugar, sweets and chocolate, and refined grains and grain products (white rice, white flour and bread, cakes, biscuits, etc.),

To avoid processed foods that may contain additives.

This means tinned, packaged, frozen, or pre-cooked foods, sweets, crisps, cakes, biscuits, fizzy drinks, etc. (Some manufacturers do now process foods without artificial additives, but even these are less beneficial than unprocessed foods.)
To avoid over-use of meat, poultry and dairy products unless they have been organically produced.
To seek out organically-grown vegetables and fruit whenever possible.
To use only cold-pressed vegetable oils and avoid frying as much as possible.
To make sure you get enough of the protective Vitamins A,C and E, plus Selenium.

If you follow these guide-lines you will not only be protecting yourself against cancer but many other dis-eases as well. Of course, this doesn't mean that you can NEVER have a packet of crisps or buy a frozen meal when you are in a rush! Just be sensible and use these suggestions as the basis for most of your eating.

ANTI-AGING FOODS

As I pointed out above, all the materials that our bodies need for repairing tissues and making new cells have to be obtained from our food. As we get older we don't absorb nutrients from our foods as well as when we were younger, nor does the process of making new cells always work as efficiently as when we were younger. The production of new cells slows down, and the cells don't always reproduce themselves accurately, so the new cells may not be perfect copies of the ones that they are intended to replace. Some scientists even think that this is the only reason why we don't live for ever.

Whether or not that is true, less efficient reproduction of cells does certainly contribute to the process of aging. It is one of the reasons that skin wrinkles, arteries harden, body organs don't work so well and even our brains become less efficient with age.

To a great extent, what I have written about cancer applies equally to aging because in both cases the process of cell formation is involved. Many of the known carcinogens are also substances that hasten the aging process, so a good first step to maintaining your health and appearance is to avoid all unnecessary chemicals in your food. Once again, this really means using natural, unprocessed foods, and looking for foods from organic sources because of the chemicals used in most commercial agriculture.

The quality of the food we eat has a very big impact on this process of cell reproduction. By "quality" I don't mean that we need to choose the most expensive foods, or buy them in the smartest shops! I mean that we need to choose foods that provide the important nutrients for cell formation. Some foods, especially fats and sugars, consist almost entirely of what nutritionists call "empty calories", meaning that they supply calories (often a very large number) without actually providing anything of real value to the body. Burgers, chips, crisps, sweets, chocolate, ice-cream, biscuits, cakes and fizzy drinks are prime examples. If you eat such foods regularly you maybe overfed but undernourished.

To stay well through and after mid-life, we need to look for foods that do the opposite: provide us with essential nutrients without piling on the calories. The guidelines set out under "Anti-Cancer Foods" apply equally to anti-aging.

Reducing our calorie intake a little also seems to contribute to longevity. When you consider that obesity contributes to heart disease, arthritis, and many other health problems this is not really surprising but there's more to it than that: when our calorie intake is reduced we absorb minerals and other nutrients more efficiently. Dr. Roy Walford, one of the leading researchers into this phenomenon, eats normally for five days of the week and fasts on the other two: he finds this easier than trying to reduce calories every day. I find the opposite easier: eating frugally Monday to Friday and having "treats" at the weekend. You may not want to do either of these things. Everybody needs to find what works best for them but if you want to pursue this approach it is important that you choose foods that are high in essential nutrients as well as low in calories. Most of the foods I have mentioned as valuable (for a variety of reasons) throughout this book fulfil these criteria. Keep the really high-calorie foods – the chips, cream sauces and chocolate gateaux – as OCCASIONAL treats.

Free radicals are involved in aging, too, and for the same reason that they increase the risk of cancer. That is, they interfere with the cells' ability to reproduce themselves properly. This can contribute to the development of arthritis and heart disease as well as cancer, and is a major cause of wrinkles and old-looking skin. Avoiding oxidized fats and making sure you get plenty of the "scavengers" will help to protect you from premature aging as well as serious illness.

Even before its role as a free radical scavenger was understood, selenium was linked to longevity. In much the same way as the absence of cancer was noticed in people living on simple, traditional diets, it was found that in certain areas of the world a significant number of people lived far longer than we consider the norm – to as much as 120 years old in some cases – and remained vigourous and healthy for most of that time. All these areas were places where selenium is abundant in the soil, and therefore in locally produced food.

I think we still have much to learn about selenium. Some women have found that it reduces hot flushes and vaginal dryness, other have found it helpful for PMT which suggest that it may be involved in making hormones as well as enzymes. My own observation is that it helps brain function: some older women who were having difficulty remembering words, names, etc. recovered all their mental agility when they took a selenium supplement regularly.

FOODS FOR YOUR SKIN AND HAIR

If you follow the general advice on nutrition in this chapter your hair and skin should look pretty good, but there are one or two more things you should know about food and outer appearance.

The appearance of your skin depends a good deal on our old friend collagen. It makes up much of the underlying layer of your skin (the dermis) and plumps out young skin, making it look smooth. As we get older and the collagen loses some of its elasticity, the skin starts to sag and wrinkle. Everything that you have read above about collagen, free radicals, vitamins and minerals (especially selenium) applies to your skin, too.

If your skin is dry or your hair lacks lustre, you may need a little more oil in your diet. Although, as we've seen, there are very good reasons to limit fats, don't overdo this to the point of eliminating them altogether. A little cold-pressed olive oil each day, in cooking or as a salad dressing will help your skin and hair as well as your general health.

Alcohol reduces the elasticity of the skin, as well as the other harmful effects discussed above, so keep it to a minimum. As one woman said "Whisky coarsens my skin as well as my soul".

SUMMING UP

It can get very confusing, can't it – all the advice in this chapter, not to mention magazines, newspapers and other books! But if you compare the advice on food for a healthy heart, for example with that on food for strong bones, or anti-cancer foods with anti-aging foods, you'll find that there is really no contradiction. There may be slight differences of emphasis, different supplements suggested to help with specific health problems, but the same basic principles recur throughout. You'll see the same items cropping up again and again in the lists of healthy foods and among the "baddies".

A healthy eating plan can be summed up like this:

Base your meals around whole grains, fresh vegetables and fruits. Add to these small amounts of protein in the form of nuts, seeds, pulses and fish (if you are not vegetarian).

Limit your intake of meat, eggs and dairy produce: you can stay perfectly healthy without these foods, but if you want to eat them do try to get them from organic producers.

Use small amounts of cold-pressed vegetable oils and reduce your intake of all other fats.

Choose cooking methods that do not destroy the nutritional content of your food. Steam vegetables lightly, or eat them raw. Throw away your frying pan and use the grill instead.

Choose foods that are as near to their natural state as possible, in other words, foods that have had little or nothing done to them between the time when they were grown and the time when you eat them.

Eat foods that are as fresh as possible – let the least possible time elapse between when they were grown and when you eat them.

Choose foods that have been organically produced whenever you can.

Avoid salt, sugar, alcohol, caffeine, colourings, flavourings and all artificial additives.

Avoid refined foods such as white rice, white flour and bread, cakes,biscuits, etc. made with them.

Eat the widest variety of foods from among those suggested.
and.......

ENJOY YOUR FOOD! It doesn't matter if you break the
rules occasionally so don't get obsessive.

If you plan your shopping, cooking and eating along these lines, add
any supplements you may need for specific health problems and make
whatever adjustments best suit your personal needs and tastes, you
will be giving yourself the best chance of staying healthy, active and
attractive for many years to come.

FOOD FOR THOUGHT

Eating simple, unprocessed foods uses far less of the world's scarce
resources than eating those which have been processed and packaged.
Much of the feed for American and European beef cattle is grown in
third-world countries on land that is desperately needed to grow
food for the local population. An acre of land producing beans will
yield ten times as much protein as an acre used for rearing cattle or
poultry. Reducing your intake of meat may save a little bit of the
rainforest from being cut down and turned into cattle ranches.

It's nice to know that what is good for our health is good for
the Planet, too.

FURTHER READING:

The Eat for Life Diet	J. Marshall & A. Heughan	*Vermilion*
Essential Supplements for Women	Reuben & Priestly	*Thorsons*
The Wright Diet	Celia Wright	*Grafton*

17

USE IT OR LOSE IT

AS I HAVE said elsewhere in this book, human bodies were designed for hard work. The earliest humans walked long distances gathering food or hunting for it. They often walked even longer distances migrating from summer encampments to winter ones. Everything they used, from tools and clothes to homes and cooking pots had to be made by hand. They had to be able to run fast enough to catch the animals they ate.....and escape from the ones that wanted to eat them! It was, quite literally, the survival of the fittest.

Even at the beginning of the twentieth century "work" meant physical work for most women. Housework was a strenuous activity with very few mechanical aids and only the better-off had any kind of transport. Women often walked long distances every day just in the process of looking after their families. We may consider life in the last decade of the 20th century a lot easier, but we pay the price of speed, convenience and comfort in terms of weaker bodies.

Exercise has become – ironically perhaps – a leisure activity but one which is essential to our long-term health.

Although our lives are very different from those of our earliest ancestors, our bodies have changed very little: the differences between ourselves and Neanderthal man and woman are mainly cosmetic. We may look prettier, but the way our hearts, muscles and other organs function is exactly the same. So, to a large extent, our bodies are under-used and this is a source of much ill-health.

Even by the mid-thirties, women who don't take any exercise are stiffer, less mobile, more likely to be constipated, have indigestion, suffer from backache and catch more colds than those who do.

By the time we are entering the menopause, an under-used body is far less resistant to dis-ease, degeneration and aging than one which has been exercised fairly regularly and the older we get,

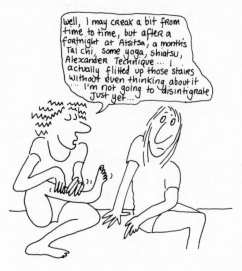

the more this becomes apparent. Women who take some kind of exercise regularly, even if it is only walking, tend to have fewer distressing symptoms during their menopause, they are more resistant to heart disease and osteoporosis,less likely to develop arthritis, their skin and hair is often in much better condition than that of their sedentary sisters.... I could go on and on.

The effects of insufficient exercise become even more apparent as we move on beyond mid-life, even in simple daily activities. Over half of women over 55 can't walk at a reasonable speed for more than a few minutes at a time, and by 65 half of all women have difficulty getting up from a chair, getting on or off a bus without help and simple tasks such as opening jars. Sadly, many people simply accept such decline as a normal part of growing older, but in fact a woman of 70 who has taken a moderate amount of exercise regularly can be as strong and supple as a sedentary woman of 40.

FIT FOR WHAT?

Exercise is often thought of as "keeping fit" and you might ask "Fit for what?" Athletes train to be fit for specific sports, dancers train to be fit for theatrical performance. Women need to train to be fit for a long life! If you are menopausal now, you are probably going to live for another 30 years or so, and if you want to make them rich, full, enjoyable years you're going to need a strong, healthy and mobile body.

WHAT KIND OF EXERCISE?

The secret of success is to choose a form of exercise you ENJOY. If you don't, you'll soon be tempted to give up. Let me tell you the story of my friend Izzy:

Izzy is in her 60's, a for-
mer ballet dancer and some-
what overweight. She went to
see her GP about an old dance
injury which had been flaring
up on and off for the past three
years. To ease her weak knee,
she tended to take her weight
as much as possible on the
other leg, and now that one
was hurting, too. The doctor
examined her knees and then
read her the riot act! "You're a
lively, intelligent woman but if
you don't do something about
it now, your body is going to
let you down while your mind
is still active", he said. Apart
from losing a stone or two, she
should swim three times a week
and ride an exercise bike. In
vain she pleaded that she hated
chlorine: "Buy some goggles"
was his reply.

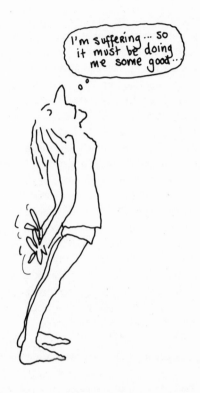

Scared into obeying, Izzy grimly set about swimming thrice
weekly, preceded by 20 minutes or so on the static bike in the gymnasium attached to the local pool. The chlorine upset her just as
much as she'd predicted, and she hated the gymnasium – there was
always loud rock music blaring, and the static bike was so boring. By
the third week, she was finding excuses to skip a session. By the
fourth week, she was sitting in my cottage in tears because she was so
ashamed of herself for giving up.

"But Izzy" I said "you know how to strengthen your knees,
without doing things you hate. What about all your ballet exercises?"

"But the doctor said I had to swim and ride that b..... bike"
she replied.

"Only because that would work your knees without putting
weight on them" I pointed out. "Which ballet exercises would have
the same effect?"

Within ten minutes she had mapped out her programme and

gone home to sort out some suitable music. She started with a sequence designed for children's dance classes, and gradually worked up to a much more demanding one. Within two months, her knees were fine and the last time I saw her, she'd just been rock climbing on Dartmoor with a group of women half her age!

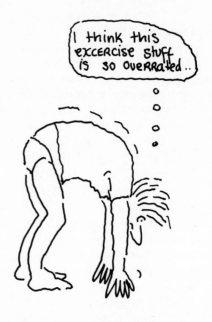

The moral of Izzy's story is that you are much more likely to stick at an exercise programme you enjoy. So if you are already taking any kind of exercise that you really like, stick with it – there's no virtue in changing, unless you need to add elements that protect you from specific problems, as outlined below and in the chapters on preventing heart disease and osteoporosis.

If you don't know what you would enjoy, start exploring all the possibilities, taking your likes and dislikes into account. Don't enrol in an aerobics class if you hate loud music, for example, or in a competitive sport if you are non-competitive by nature. If you like the great outdoors, look for an outdoor activity, if you are a loner by nature, find something you can do alone. There is a great deal to be said, though, for classes where a teacher can keep an eye on you and make certain you are not doing anything incorrectly which could damage your body in any way. Adult education classes, health clubs and private classes are available almost everywhere and all should allow you to take a sample class before you decide whether to enrol. In many places, there are classes especially for older people. If they don't cater for the activity you think you would enjoy, make sure the class you would like to join is not beyond your present ability. Talk to the teacher beforehand about any physical problems you may have, and say honestly if you are out of condition or have not exercised for a long time. If you have any major health problems, talk to your doctor first. You may be advised to take things gently to start with but, with very few exceptions, your doctor will confirm that any exercise is better for your health than no exercise at all.

If you don't know where to start, here are a few ideas to whet your appetite:

Walking, running, jogging, skipping, dancing (ballet, contemporary, tap, folk, jazz, ballroom, etc.) swimming and pool exercises, tennis, badminton, archery, fencing, golf, riding, cycling, sailing, skating, weight training, gymnastics, "keep-fit" in all its varieties, tai-chi, judo, karate, yoga.

If you have not been in the habit of taking exercise, yoga is an ideal choice because it is non-competitive and the teacher will discourage you from trying to do anything that is beyond your present ability. As you grow stronger you can do more.

Whatever form of exercise you choose, don't be impatient with yourself. It may take longer to notice any changes in your body than when you were in your 20's or 30's. Our muscles become less elastic as oestrogen levels decrease, so it will take longer for you to see outer changes such as a firmer tummy, for example. But do persevere, because your body will benefit right from the beginning: every time you exercise you strengthen your heart and circulation, your bones and muscles, your lymphatic system (helping to prevent fluid retention) and your whole body. The condition of your skin and hair will improve and you will quite likely find that you sleep better and, conversely, that you have more energy. It's not only your body that will feel better, either: exercise influences the chemicals in our brain that affect mood and you will almost certainly feel brighter as a result.

To be of any long-term benefit, exercise needs to be regular. A little every day is better, and safer, than saving it all up until the weekend. The minimum that will give you long-term "health insurance" is 20 minutes every other day, and it is better if one of the sessions is an hour long.

If you join a class of any kind, or a gymnasium or health club, the instructor will build in a warm-up period at the beginning of your exercise session and a cooling-down sequence at the end. If you choose to exercise independently, it is really important to allow a few minutes for this at the beginning and end of each session to avoid muscle strains and stiffness. Here is a simple warm-up sequence, starting from your head and working down to your feet. Repeat each of the suggested movements ten to twelve times.

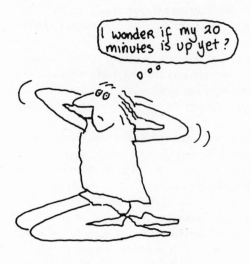

Drop your chin on to your chest and slowly roll your head from side to side.

Make circles with your shoulders by lifting them up towards your ears as far as they will go, pulling them backwards and then letting them drop down again. After 10 or 12 circles, try doing this in the opposite direction.

Swing both arms in big circles, then change directions and repeat.

Keeping your hips still, turn the upper half of your body from side to side. Do this fairly slowly and gently and DON'T try to increase the movement by swinging your arms.

Make big circles with your hips as if you were swinging a hula-hoop.Repeat in the opposite direction.

Bend your knees as far as they will comfortably go and press up again.

Hold on to something and swing one leg backwards and forwards, then the other leg.

Still holding on, lift one foot off the ground and move it in circles from the ankle. Repeat in the other direction and then with the other foot.

This sequence is also very good for maintaining or increasing your general mobility so it is good to do it regularly even on days when you are not doing any other exercise. It only takes a few minutes and gets all the major joints moving, which is an important consideration as we get older.

If you feel any form of exercise is beyond you, just walk. Walking is the one form of exercise that everybody can do, regardless of age or state of health. Walk a little bit each day and try to increase the time and distance bit by bit. As you get used to it, try to walk a little faster, too: it will benefit your heart.

Within the above guidelines you can make slight changes of emphasis depending on your particular health needs, so in the rest of this chapter I shall describe more specifically the kind of exercise that will strengthen your bones, reduce your risk of heart disease, alleviate backache and help prevent or treat prolapse of the womb.

EXERCISE FOR A HEALTHY HEART

Exercise for a healthy heart needs to raise your pulse rate – in other words, it needs to make your heart beat a little faster. You should also feel warmer, maybe sweating a little, and slightly "puffed" (though only slightly – if you are really out of breath you may have been working too hard for your present state of fitness). Such exercise is called aerobic exercise (which can be confusing because it has nothing to do with jumping about in shiny leotards!) or you may hear doctors and exercise teachers referring to it as cardio-vascular exercise. Cycling, running, most kinds of dancing, weight training, jogging, really brisk walking, tennis, martial arts and so forth are all good aerobic exercise. Swimming is, too, if done fast and continuously.

Whichever you choose, be sure to include a warm-up at the beginning and a cooling-down period of gentler exercise at the end of your session. If you are working with a teacher in a class, it should be structured to include this. If you exercise independently, use the sequence described above, or something similar.

If you are unfit or already have any kind of heart problem or high blood pressure, start with something gentle and talk to your doctor and to the class teacher beforehand to be sure that you are not taking any health risks. But please believe me when I say that taking no exercise at all is a far greater risk.

EXERCISE FOR STRONG BONES

Exercise must involve some effort against the pull of gravity if it is to have a strengthening effect on your bones. (Astronauts lose bone-mass during space flights however much they move about because the element of gravity is absent.) Such forms of exercise are some-times called "bone-loading" and include walking, running, jogging, dancing, skipping, weight-training, gymnastics, athletics, tennis, bad-minton, martial arts, tai-chi and yoga.

Swimming is not so effective because the weight of the body is supported by the water. Cycling and exercise bikes are good cardiovascular exercise but do not help to strengthen the bones of your legs and hips because most of your body-weight is supported by the saddle. Weight-carrying exercise for the bones of the legs and hips is particularly important because fractures of the hip (or neck of the femur) are one of the commonest and most serious results of osteoporosis. So if your main exercise is swimming or cycling, it is good to add a session of dance, yoga, tai-chi, etc. at least once a week or, at very least, an hour's brisk walking.

If you are already suffering from bone-loss, exercise can slow down or even halt the progress of disease, and there is a growing amount of evidence, especially from work being done in Israel, that it can even replace some of the lost bone-mass. Of course, you will need to embark on any exercise programme very gently and carefully and with expert supervision. Anything which involves repeated impact, such as running, jogging or skipping would be positively dangerous and could lead to fractures. Take advice from the doctor or therapist who is treating you and talk to any class teacher before you try anything.

EXERCISE FOR A STRONG AND SUPPLE BACK

Backache is misery, and it affects most people at some point in their lives, but tends to be a more persistent problem as we get older. This can be due to "wear and tear" on the spinal vertebrae, to specific disease affecting the bones, such as arthritis or osteoporosis, but more often than not it is not the bones but the muscles that surround and support them that are the source of the pain. Fortunately, muscles respond very well to exercise, and there are some easy exercises that greatly reduce back pain and often get rid of it altogether. Most of these are based on yoga, and although it is generally inadvisable to practise yoga alone unless you have already had some tuition from a trained teacher, these back exercises are so helpful and so unlikely to do any harm, that I am going to describe several of them in detail. All of them are done on the floor, either lying or kneeling, so it will help if you have a yoga mat, rug or folded blanket to work on.

Spinal rolls
Lying flat on your back, bend up your knees and stretch your arms out on the floor on either side, so that they are in line with your shoulders. (Diag. 2) Allow your knees to slowly fall towards the floor on your right and at the same time, turn your head gently to the left.

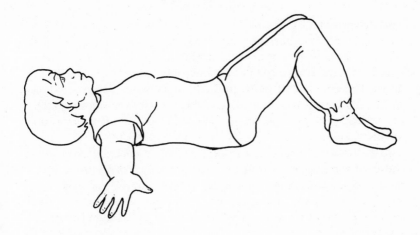

Diagram 2.

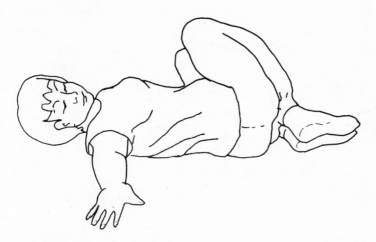

Diagram 3.

Bring your knees and head back to their starting positions still nice and slowly – then drop your knees to the left as you roll your head to the right (Diag. 3). Don't forget to breathe easily as you drop your knees to each side in turn ten, twelve or more times. It doesn't matter if your knees don't get as far as the floor, so don't force them down. Try to keep both shoulders and both hips on the floor.

The Pelvic Tilt

Start in the same position but with your arms near your sides (Diag.4). Breathe in and as you breathe out, press the lower part of your back hard against the floor, using only your tummy muscles to do so. The little hollow between the floor and your waist should disappear and your pelvis tilt forward (Diag. 5). Hold this position for a few seconds, then breathe in as you relax. DON'T lift your bottom off the floor at all, and DON'T let your legs "help". If you find it hard to isolate the tummy muscles, imagine somebody dropping a packet of frozen peas on your tummy and those muscles involuntarily tightening as a reaction to the cold and the surprise. To start with, try doing this eight times, having a little rest and doing another eight. As you get stronger, try doing two sets of ten, and then two sets of twelve.

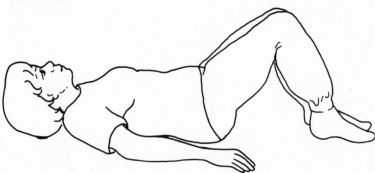

Diagram 4.

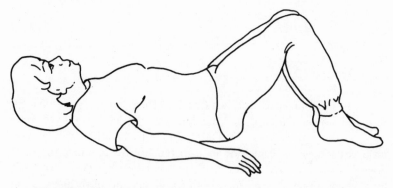

Diagram 5.

The Little Bridge

Start in the same position as for the Pelvic Tilt. (Diag.4) This time, you are going to lift your bottom off the floor. Press your arms and hands gently against the floor as you lift your hips up off the ground. It doesn't matter if you

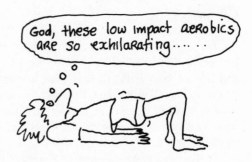

only get them a few inches off the floor: it is the effort of doing so that will benefit your body. As you get stronger, you can try to lift your hips higher. Make sure you keep your shoulders firmly on the floor. Hold this position (Diag. 6) for a few moments, then come back to your starting position by rolling your back down, vertebra by vertebra from the top downwards. Do this three or four times in all.

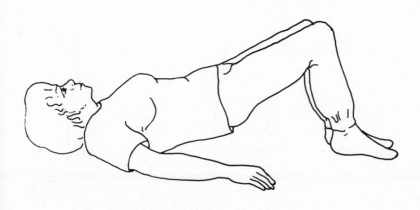

Diagram 6.

Cat Stretch

For this one, start by kneeling on all fours. (Diag.7) Your hands should be directly underneath your shoulders, and your knees should be directly underneath your hips. Breathe in, gently lift your head and hollow your back, so that your bottom sticks up and your waist drops down (Diag.8) Now breathe out as you drop your head, tuck your bottom under and arch your back like a cat (Diag. 9) Alternate these two positions eight or ten times , moving slowly and smoothly all the time.

This exercise really helps to prevent back pain and stiffness and gives real relief if your back is already stiff and painful so try to do it every day, or even several times a day. It's especially useful to practise the Cat Stretch after you have been sitting for a long time.

Any exercises that tone the tummy muscles will help low back pain as well because your muscles form a continuous band around the front and back of your body, so weak muscles that allow your tummy to sag at the front will put extra strain on your lower back. Just thinking about your tummy muscles and pulling them in for a few seconds several times a day will help.

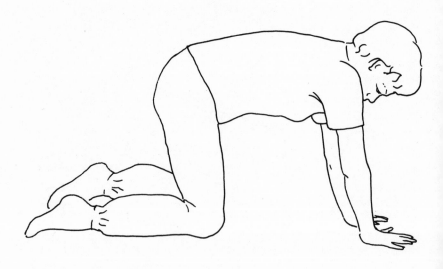

Diagram 7.

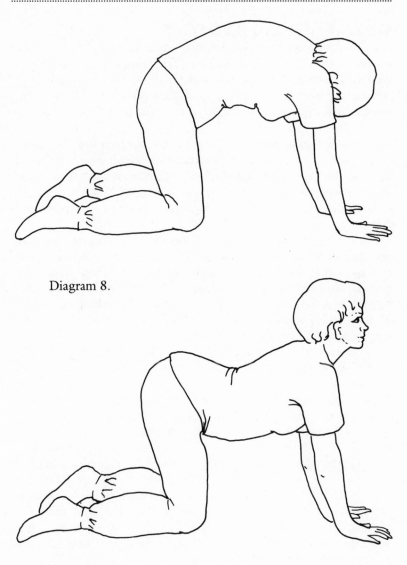

Diagram 8.

Diagram 9.

Poor posture is often a cause of backache, so try standing and walking with your pelvis gently tucked forward. If you have really bad back pain, it would be a good idea to see an osteopath or chiropractor before starting on any exercises.

STAYING STRONG AND SEXY

O.K., I admit I only put that bit in to make sure you read on! The exercises I am going to describe here WILL heighten pleasure if you are sexually active, but what is far more important is that they help to prevent and even correct prolapse of the womb. All older women, whether sexually active or not, need to know about these exercises and practise them regularly.

I'm referring to pelvic floor exercises, which are sometimes called Kegel exercises after the Canadian obstetrician who popularised them in the West, although Indian women have used these techniques for thousands of years. If you have had children, you will probably have been taught these exercises as part of your post-natal care.

To strengthen your pelvic floor muscles, imagine that you need to pass urine but can't get to a toilet immediately: squeeze your muscles firmly as though to stop yourself urinating. Hold the squeeze while you count to three, relax, then the repeat the squeeze. If you find it difficult to identify which muscles you should be using, try this initially when you are actually on the toilet and try to stop your urine in mid-stream.

Once you have got the hang of this exercise you can try increasing the time that you hold the squeeze, until you can hold for a count of ten before you relax. Also, try squeezing and relaxing quickly without any hold or pause in between. As your pelvic floor muscles get stronger and you get more skillful, you may be able to isolate different areas and try squeezing the muscles around your vagina, anus and urethra (the opening from the bladder) alternately.

To be effective, these exercises need to be repeated dozens of times each day, some people advise as many as 200 repetitions but you can do them anywhere, at any time and nobody will know what you are doing. Do them while are waiting at the bus stop, doing the washing-up or watching a film. Try them lying down at first, but remember that they are more effective when you have to work against gravity and do at least some repetitions sitting or standing each day. Don't try to do 100 or more at one session – divide them into several shorter sets.

Gynaecologists usually teach these exercises in isolation, but they are more effective if you strengthen the muscles of the surrounding areas as well. Try crossing your legs and pressing your thighs hard against each other. Do this ten times, then change legs and do ten more. Clench and unclench your buttock muscles ten or twelve times, several times a day. Pull in your tummy muscles whenever you think of it ..... but make sure that you DO think of it often! Your abdominal muscles really help to support your uterus in position.

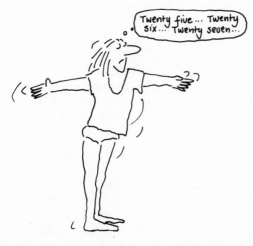

As well as preventing prolapse, pelvic floor exercises help to prevent and cure urinary incontinence. If you leak a little urine when you laugh or cough, practising these exercises regularly will almost always correct the problem.

Finally, the "Strong and sexy" heading was no joke. Exercising the pelvic area regularly increases the local blood supply (as does exercise for any part of the body) and this helps to keep the walls of the vagina strong, elastic and moist. This will contribute to your personal comfort and well-being whether you are in a sexual relationship or not. If you are sexually active, learning to contract or relax these muscles at will can increase your enjoyment of sex and your partner's, too.

FURTHER READING:

Bone Loading	Simkin & Alayon	*Prion*
Fit to be Fifty	Samantha Lee	*Chapmans*
The Ageless Body	Chris Griscom	*Light Institute Press*
Yoga for Women	N. Phelan & M. Volin	*Arrow*

18

LOOKING AFTER YOUR FEELINGS

IN THE LAST few chapters we have examined at some length at the various ways you can look after your body during and after menopause. But menopause is not only a physical event, and there are times when we need to look after our feeling selves as well.

Of course, the two are not separate: whatever affects our hearts and mind affects our bodies, too, and vice versa.

We looked briefly, in Chapter 2, at some of the emotional trauma that can affect us during our middle years, and at the fact that while some of them are directly connected to the advent of menopause, others simply happen around the same time. The loss of a partner through divorce, separation or death is a fairly common experience, and our own mid-life is often the time when our parents or other older relatives and friends die. These things could happen to us at any time, they have nothing to do with menopause, but when they coincide with it our natural grief, hurt and anger may be intensified because we feel insecure during this period of change and transition or because we are not feeling well physically.

If this happens to you, please don't bottle up your grief. To go inwards, almost hugging your grief to yourself, is part of the process of mourning. You need time to mourn, but you also need eventually to move out of this inward-looking phase. Express your sadness to other members of your family, talk to your friends, your children, even your grandchildren if you have any. It's much easier for them to offer you comfort if you acknowledge that you need it.

It may help, too, to go outside the circle of your family and friends and talk to a bereavement counsellor who can help you work through the mixed emotions that often follow the death of somebody close.

Divorce or separation can give rise to even more complex emotions: loss, anger, abandonment, failure and rejection are just

some of them and here again, a counsellor can help you to understand and resolve them. Don't struggle on alone when there is help
available. On top of the emotional trauma of a broken relationship,
there are often problems of a strictly practical nature, like lack of
finance, a forced house-move, coping with children alone, difficulties
around the question of custody and access and much more which
add to the mental stress. So be kind to yourself and ask for help when
you need it, whether it is a shoulder to cry on, a listening ear, two or
three friends to help you heave packing cases or somebody to have
the kids for a few hours while you unwind. Many of us are so used to
looking after everyone else's needs that we get out of the habit of
looking after our own.

Women who have done little else but look after other people's
needs for 20 years or so are often the ones who suffer most emotional
distress during mid-life. However much one rejects the concept that
woman's only true work is child-bearing and child-rearing, many
women do experience a great sense of loss and emptiness when the
last child leaves home. The more exclusively they have devoted themselves to the wife-and-mother role the more likely this is. Mothers
who have also worked outside their home, kept up hobbies or
pursued other outside interests are less vulnerable to depression at
this point in their lives.

If you are finding it difficult to come to terms with a child
leaving home, it might help to use the affirmation "I love you
enough to let you go". Write it on a card and put it somewhere
where you will see it often, and try saying the words either aloud or
in your head several times each day, and think of your child on the
brink of adulthood as you do so. Imagine saying this directly to your
child, and perhaps you will find at some point that you can do so in
actual fact. It can help too, to remind yourself that all the love and
care you have given to this child have prepared him or her well to
become independent and that it would not help the child at all to
stay dependent on you any longer. Jung says that a wise parent
knows when to hold a child close and when to loosen the ties.

For some women emotional trauma stems from a totally
opposite cause: if you have not had children the physical fact of not
ovulating any more can have a poignant finality about it. This is
especially painful if you have tried to have babies and have not con-
ceived, or have miscarried or had a stillborn child, but some women
who have children already feel great sadness at this time if they have

remarried or are in a new relationship and would have liked to have children with their present partner. It is just as important to express this grief as it is when a loved person dies. Really acknowledge the regret you feel for those lost babies, and perhaps make a ceremony to mourn them. It is only when you allow your grief into the open that you can heal it.

Loneliness can become a major issue for older women living alone. It affects women who are divorced or bereaved and those who have never married or entered into other long-term relationship. Single women who have cared for an invalid parent can feel very bereft when that parent dies, because the responsibility of caring has often prevented them having much social life. It can be difficult to make new friendships, but please do try to do so, and to stay close to the friends you already have. Friends are important for our emotional health throughout our life, but never more so than as we get older. People with friends actually live longer! A study in America found that people with strong social bonds (lovers, friends, clubs, organizations, etc.) had a lower mortality rate than people who were more isolated, irrespective of age.

Although many older women do re-marry or form new relationships, we have to be realistic and remember that women, statistically, live longer than men and there will always be more lone women than lone men. Pinning all your hopes on remarrying or finding a new lover can prevent you enjoying the positive aspects of being on your own, especially the freedom to do whatever you like, whenever you like. If you are alone, relish that freedom, but at the same time try to build up a network of good friends for mutual support.

Petra is in her 60's and lives in a country town. "I spent most of my life in London, but when my youngest son left home I bought a house on the outskirts of a small village. At first it seemed idyllic and I was too busy doing up the house and garden to notice I hadn't made any real friends but after a while I realised that the local community was very closed and nobody in the village shared my interests. After a couple of years I was so lonely and depressed I moved again to a busy market town. I've been here four years now, and I have a big network of friends in the town and the surrounding villages, far more, in fact than when I lived in London. I'm always meeting somebody for lunch or coffee and some of us share lifts to Bristol for the theatre and concerts, or go to London for the day to see an exhibition. If I'm fed up with my own company indoors, I only need walk up the High Street and I'll almost certainly meet six people I know! It's marvellous."

I think it took some courage on Petra's part to move house a second time, but it was clearly better for her than staying put and being lonely. What Petra does not include in this part of her account (her story was too long to include in its entirety) is that she sought help from a counsellor when the feeling of isolation made her really depressed: "Living out in the sticks, I had to drive 40 miles to see Jill, but it happened to be a beautiful drive and I simply allowed the journey to become part of my therapy. When I first thought about moving, Jill helped me to clarify my motives. We made a list together of what I hoped to gain by doing that,to be sure I wasn't "running away" but doing something positive to make my life better and I think one reason I have got so much out of my new life here is that the counselling helped me to get certain priorities sorted out."

As I have already suggested, skilled counselling is of immense value to anybody who is suffering mental or emotional stress whatever the cause. Don't think that whatever is troubling you is too trivial to warrant taking a counsellor's time: if you are in distress, for whatever reason, you deserve help. Counsellors are trained to be non-judgemental and will not "blame" you for anything that you may be thinking or feeling, or for anything that you have done or not done.

It can happen that stressful events such as bereavement, divorce or parting from a child give rise to even more emotional distress than the event itself would seem to warrant, or a period of depression goes on for a very long time. If you are seriously distressed, whatever the reason, it may be that going a little deeper than counselling and seeking some form of psychotherapy would be wise. I have said before, but I will stress again, that you do not have to be mentally ill to benefit from psychotherapy. I know that some people feel that there is a certain stigma attached to entering therapy, so I will "come out" and state unequivocally that I have experienced great personal benefit from therapy (psychosynthesis) which helped me through a period of emotional distress and enabled me to make some important changes in my life. I think I am a happier and stronger person because of it.

Therapy can support people through a time of transition and menopause is a time of transition for every woman, whatever the other circumstances in her life may be.

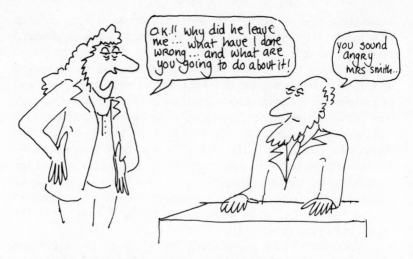

Some therapists use writing, painting, drawing, sound, movement or role-play as part of the work they do with clients and these are also ways in which you can help yourself, whether or not you choose to work with a therapist as well. Dance workshops, drama-therapy, art-therapy, creative writing, etc., are all vehicles through which we can release emotion. Some of these, especially writing and drawing or painting we can do alone,too.

A particularly effective self-help method is known as Creative Journal keeping. The Creative Journal is a book you can write in

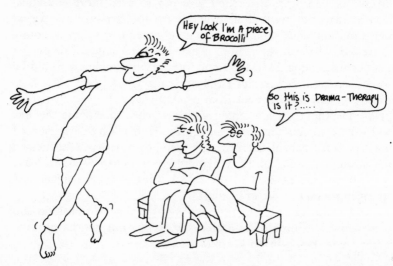

146

every day, or just when you have something you need to express. It is quite different from the kind of diary that goes "Got up at 7.00, fed the cat, burnt the toast........". In this kind of journal you write whatever is on your mind, what you are feeling at that moment, record your dreams and fantasies or just whatever you want to put in it. You can draw – and it doesn't matter at all whether your drawings are "good": they are simply a way of expressing and exploring your feelings. If you are feeling absolutely ghastly, you might colour a whole page black, or write "YUCK!" in huge letters, or draw a cartoon figure that represents yourself looking glum...whatever works best for you. You can use coloured pens to write different thoughts or draw boxes round individual words. It may sound trivial when described like this, but it is fun, and it works.

Jackie is somebody who tried creative journal keeping:

"I came across the idea of Creative Journal when somebody gave a talk about it locally. I was quite ill at the time, and I used my journal to explore my feelings about my illness and not being in control of my body. I had a lot of strange dreams at that time which I recorded in my journal and being able to read them later, sometimes several days or weeks after they occurred, often helped me to make sense of them. Later, I used the journal as quite a fun thing, drawing cartoons about everyday occurrences and the people in my life. When I split up with my boyfriend in rather explosive circumstances, I filled page after page with "revenge" cartoons in which I was clobbering him with a huge mallet and so on! I laugh my head off when I look back through the book, but I realise now that I got over the break-up remarkably quickly considering how traumatic it was at the time, and I think the journal work helped me do so."

I keep a creative journal, too (though it gets rather neglected when I'm writing a book like this!) and can vouchsafe for its effectiveness as a way of dealing with all kinds of feelings.

You might well invent a method that works equally well for you.

Other ways of looking after your feelings include making sure you get enough time to yourself, and enough time spent with really good friends, learning to relax, learning meditation, reminding yourself that you matter as much as any of the people around you, not always putting other people first, getting enough hugs, giving yourself "treats", listening to beautiful music and anything else that you find nurturing. Treat yourself to a massage once in a while, have a scented bath, buy yourself a bunch of flowers or a new book, stand in the middle of a field and scream your rage to the sky, or just stand there and enjoy all the sights and sounds around you.

Remember that your mind and body are intimately connected and that mental stress or emotional distress can make menopausal problems worse, just as physical pain, lack off sleep or continual discomfort can make non-physical problems harder to cope with. You are a whole person embracing mind, body and spirit, and you owe it to yourself to look after every part of that whole.

FURTHER READING:

The Creative Journal, The Art of Finding Yourself	Lucia Capacchione	*Newcastle Pub Co. Inc*
You Can Heal Your Life	Louise Hay	*Eden Grove*
Positively Single	Vera Peifer	*Element*
Meditations for Women Who Do Too Much	Anne Wilson Schaef	*Harper Collins*
Life-Cycle Celebrations for Women	Marge Sears	*Twenty-third Publications*

PART III
A CHANGE FOR THE BETTER

This part of the book is about the opportunities that are waiting for you. It is about all the wonderful things that older women have done and that you can do, too! I hope you find it inspiring.

19

RITES OF PASSAGE

ONE OF THE reasons that menopause can seem mysterious and threatening is that we talk about it so little. Women pass through a period of major change with little or no opportunity to share their experiences and certainly no formal way to mark the event. We have ceremonies for birth and death and for marriage, but no way to celebrate two of the most important transitions in a woman's life: puberty and menopause.

Earlier cultures knew better. They marked these milestones with rituals: sometimes in closed circles that excluded the menfolk, sometimes in their families or larger social group. The few non-urbanised societies that survive still preserve their old traditions and there is evidence that the women in such societies move through menopause more gracefully than their civilised sisters. Native American women, for example, become members of the Grand-mothers' Lodge when they have had no more menstrual periods for fourteen moons. The Grandmothers are respected for their wisdom and become the teachers of the younger women.

Perhaps we need to re-invent ritual, in ways that feel appro-priate to us as twentieth-century women. With no tradition or tribal memories to draw on, we are free to create new ceremonies with as much poetry, symbolism, emotion, pride or humour as we wish.

For example, one group of women organised an evening picnic. They took a few bottles of wine, got a little tipsy, sang songs late into the night and made a bonfire of sanitary towels. In doing so, they may have sown the seeds of a new tradition, for I have since heard of several other groups or individuals doing something similar.

Jesssica, on the day of her early retirement, made a ritual bonfire of papers associated with the job she had just left. For her, freedom to pursue other interests felt more important than freedom from monthly periods.

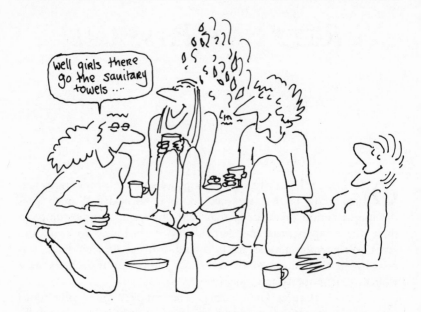

Kay turned her fiftieth birthday party into a celebration of the fertile years that were coming to their natural conclusion. She pinned up photos of her children, from their births to adulthood and gathered them all together to reminisce about everything from the first tooth to the first love affair. They brought their partners and some of them brought their own children, too. Her two sons did all the cooking for the party – a small recognition of the many, many meals she had made them over the years.

A ceremony may need to acknowledge aspects of our earlier life that we are sorry to leave behind. For example, some women feel that the end of menstruation is an occasion to be mourned rather than celebrated: this is especially true for women who are childless, or who would have liked to have another child. Mourning also needs ritual. It is important to acknowledge the grief and a simple ceremony is a very powerful way of doing so.

Eva wrote a letter to the children she had never had, her friend Sue wrote a poem and together they buried the documents and laid flowers on the spot, as if on a tiny grave. Both of them wept a lot, but they felt that expressing their sorrow in this way had left them better able to move on into a different phase of life.

Laura suffered deep depression in her late fifties for which she sought help from a psychotherapist. She was a distinguished academic, considered a leader in her particular field but now, approaching retirement, she resented the very success which she felt had isolated her and taken up her time so totally that she had not pursued her other interests, particularly music. Her therapist created a ritual for Laura which included acknowledging and honouring all her past achievements before saying goodbye to them. The ceremony helped Laura to feel good about what she had done in the past and plan for an active, creative retirement.

Elizabeth made a totem that represented her adult self. She stuck a sturdy twig into a base of modelling clay and decorated it with objects that symbolised various aspects of her life: a dried flower for her love of gardening, a needle for sewing, a spoon for all the mouths she'd fed, scraps of curtain fabric from the three houses she had made home, a pen, a paintbrush and finally a beautiful white feather which, she said, stood for her spiritual aspirations.

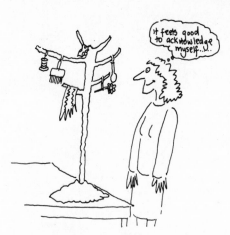

So, you see, ceremony can take any form you like. All that matters is that it means something to you. If you would like to create a rite of passage for yourself, write down all the things about menopause or getting older that you are pleased about: it might be anything from "No more pre-menstrual tension" to "I'm looking forward to retiring soon".

Then write down anything you are sorry to loose: maybe "I'm sad that I can't have a baby with my new partner", or whatever is true in your own life.

Don't forget to honour everything you have already contributed to the world. Whether your life so far has been filled with nappy changing or computer programming, teaching maths or selling shoes, doesn't matter: whatever you have done has been of value, maybe in ways that you'll never know, so find a way to recognise that in your ceremony.

Next, decide whether you want your ritual to be private, or shared with a few close friends, or a bigger group, or with your family.

Finally, draw on your own feminine creativity to decide what would be the most appropriate way to symbolise your time of transition: do you want to have a party, meditate in silence, paint a picture, dance or sing? Whatever it is, do it wholeheartedly. It will help you move on into the next stage of your life.

FURTHER READING:

Life-Cycle Celebrations for Women	Marge Sears	*Twentythird Publications*
Mother Wit	Diane Mariechild	*The Crossing Press*
She Lives!	Judith Laura	*The Crossing Press*

20

GOING BACK TO SCHOOL

WE ARE ENCOURAGED to study when we are very young, whether we like it or not, but for many of us, study goes to the bottom of the priority list once we become immersed in the "serious" business of adult life. Ironically, the years when society makes it easiest for us to study, by providing grants, educational facilities and overt approval of such "serious" activity, are not always the time when we want to take advantage of all that is on offer. We may feel that earning lots of money, having babies or travelling to India are much better options, however much our anxious parents urge us to finish our "A" levels, go to university or whatever.

Conversely, some young people who would like to stay longer at school and go on to further education are discouraged by their parents, sometimes because there is a real need for the young person to bring additional income into the family and sometimes because there is no family tradition of higher education.

The most typical time for returning to education is the mid-forties, though I have met wonderful women in their eighties studying everything from art to yoga.

The significance of the mid-forties is that this is a time when children may be leaving home, or are at least old enough not to need constant care and supervision. For many mothers, this is the first opportunity to study that they have had since their own childhood.

Deciding what, where and how you would like to study will depend on many factors, such as whether you are doing it "for fun" or as a stepping stone towards a career change or qualification, whether you like studying alone or would rather be in a class with other people, how much time you have available and - the bottom line in some cases – what classes are available in your chosen subject and in your area.

For most people the most accessible are the adult education classes run by local authorities. Don't turn up your nose at them. Even though the classes are sometimes in uninspiring surroundings, the range of courses on offer in some areas is staggering. Sports, dance, music, art, all kinds of crafts, cookery, languages, computer studies, first aid: even in the small country town where I live all these, and more, are on offer and in larger towns and cities the choice is even greater and if you add in the classes organised by the Workers Educational Association (WEA) which often shares facilities with the local authority classes, the scope is even greater. Almost every local education authority offers G.C.S.E. courses for adults in a variety of subjects.....well, why not? I took "A" levels at the same time as my 18yr old daughter!

If you want to go beyond "A" level, some adult education centres are able to offer university extension courses, and, of course there is the Open University. The OU is justifiably proud of the number of older people who have obtained degrees via their courses, though by no means all their students are working towards degrees. There are also many OU courses you can study for your own pleasure and enrichment. At usually takes about 5 years to complete a degree course, and it does require plenty of motivation and discipline to study at home though you will have support from your tutor and contact with tutors and other students at Summer Schools.

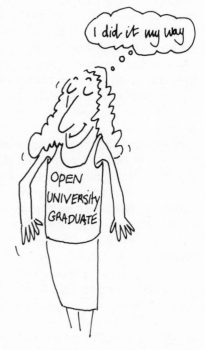

This combination of home study and contact with tutors and other students is not exclusive to the Open University, though it is probably the success of the OU that has made this form of study academically acceptable. Once upon a time, correspondence courses were rather looked down upon. Now they are accepted as a valid way of studying and are often a welcome option for women at mid-life who still have family responsibilities and/or demanding jobs, but want to study something new. For the past 11 years I have taught an aromatherapy course that is organised on similar lines to the OU and some of the most committed and successful students have been the women of forty-plus.

The National Extension College is another organization offering a very wide choice of courses (well over 100) at all levels from leisure study, through G.C.S.E. to degree level.

Home study courses are available covering a huge variety of subjects, from journalism to painting and sculpture, so if there are no facilities in your area to study the subject of your choice, or if the flexibility of studying this way would suit you and your lifestyle, you can probably find a course to fill your needs. Many of the best courses are accredited by the Council for the Accreditation of Correspondence Courses (C.A.C.C.)

Before embarking on home study, ask yourself these questions:

Do I enjoy working by myself? Can I arrange enough quiet, uninterrupted time at home to study effectively? Will my partner/children/flatmates, etc. support my decision and respect the time I set aside for study? If the answer to any of these is "no" it may be that this is not the best way for you to study, though if the only problem is likely to be a lack of a quiet place or time in which to work, I do know a couple of determined women who have got around this by going to the public library or to a friend's home to read and write.

Doreen is one of these women. Although she was studying at local adult education classes she had a lot of homework to do, and some of her problems were similar to those of students on correspondence courses:

"When I was 41 I wanted to study for a degree but I found that I needed two "A" levels in subjects other than the ones I'd done at 18. So I enroled for "A" level classes at my local adult education institute. My kids were in their teens and studying for exams themselves, and were mostly pretty co-operative but my husband was totally unsupportive. The only place I could write essays, etc. was on the kitchen table after dinner was cleared away but he often came home late when the rest of us had finished eating, and if he saw I was studying he would not attempt to get his own meal, even if that only meant lifting it out of the oven. Later in the year, as the exams approached, he got even more disruptive, and would play loud music or invite friends home and talk noisily over my head. For the last few weeks before the exams I went to a friend's house twice a week to do my revision. I did pass, with good grades, but his behaviour did nothing to help our already shaky marriage, and we split up not long after. I postponed applying for my degree course while I sorted out a divorce, selling the house and all that, but I finally got to college when I was 45 and got my BA at the age of 48."

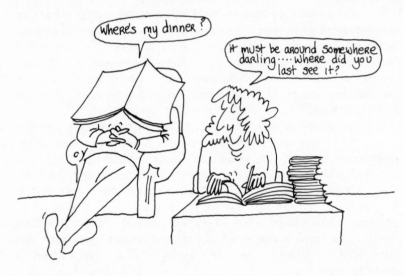

Returning to study full time is, of course, an even bigger undertaking but one that many older women have found immensely satisfying. For some of them, this has fulfilled a long-held wish, often to study something they were unable to when younger. For others, the return to study has been to pursue a new interest – after all, we change and our interests change and the passions of our teens and twenties may not be those of our forties or fifties. But the most frequent reason for re-entering full time education is to facilitate a change of career. Full time study is sometimes the only way to obtain a training or qualification needed to make such a change.

Questions concerning household arrangements and support from family may need even more thought and for many women there are financial implications that need working out in advance. If you are in a full-time job, can you manage without that income for three or four years? Will you be able to get a grant for the course you wish to take? (Few education authorities will now give grants to students over 50.)

If you have children still at home, you'll need to think through your domestic arrangements well in advance. If they are young enough to need taking to and from school how will their hours and yours dovetail? Will you need to pay somebody to take care of them after school until you get home? Most teenage children are able to put simple meals together or reheat something you have made beforehand, do their own ironing and take a share of other chores, and if you have been a working mother, they may already be used to doing so but it pays to talk through proposed arrangements with them very carefully. If they have been used to you taking care of them in obvious, physical ways, such as cooking, they may need re-assurance that you love them just as much now that you are not filling that role exclusively (and the same goes for husbands and partners). Older children, though, can be really good allies in that they understand only too well the pressures involved in reading, revision and getting essays in on time!

The problems involved in caring for and maintaining a good relationship with children are magnified for single parents but, despite the difficulties, single mothers form a sizeable proportion of mature women students. This is often because divorce has left them with a very low income and retraining is a way for them to eventually increase their earning capacity.

Some colleges offer part-time courses, for perhaps two or three days a week, as an alternative to full time, and these are often designed with the mature student in mind. Studying this way may mean taking up to five years to complete a course that would last for three years if you attended full time. Where this option is available it is worth thinking through the pros and cons very carefully before applying. Would you be willing to postpone the day when you walk out with your BA or your HND in Engineering in order to have some free days each week for shopping and essential chores, or are you prepared to put up with the inconvenience and, often, exhaustion, of cramming your entire domestic responsibility into evenings and weekends in return for reaching your goal in the shortest possible time?

The challenges involved in returning to full time study are not only domestic and financial: many mature students will not have done any serious study for 20 years or more and it is not always easy to make the switch from housewife/mother/employee to student. Sometimes, studying part-time for a while first is a way of easing the transition. You might want to study some subjects at evening classes first, like Doreen who we met above, or find out whether there are any "Access" or "Returning to Study" courses available in your subject area. These usually run for one or two days a week for a year and are designed specifically for people who have not studied for some years. Many colleges accept completion of such a course as an alternative to "A" levels for mature students seeking entry.

If you are thinking about applying for a college or university course, it is a good idea to find out roughly what proportion of each year's intake are mature students, also to bear in mind that "mature" in this context means anybody over 25! Don't be afraid to ask the admissions officer, or tutors you meet at an interview, how many older people are likely to be on your course. And ask

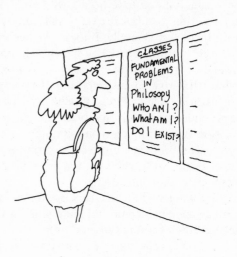

yourself whether you want to spend a major part of the next three years with fellow-students who are young enough to be your children! Generally speaking, age differences are soon forgotten, but I met one woman who made herself an outsize badge saying "I am not your mother" when the younger students began treating her as if she was!

If you want to study for mental stimulation and your own pleasure, rather than as a means to getting a qualification or preparing for a career change, you might like to investigate the University of the Third Age (U3A). This is an organization run by and for people over 50, providing classes in a huge range of subjects. U3A originated in France 21 years ago, and the English equivalent is celebrating its tenth birthday this year (1993). It is not a "university" in the usual

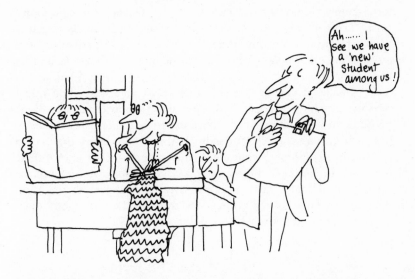

sense of the word, (unlike the OU, for example) in that it does not prepare students for degrees or any other qualification. Classes are purely recreational, and members of each local group decide what classes they would like. Teachers are all drawn from the local membership so if, for example, some members of a branch ask for French conversation and there is an experienced French speaker in that group, a class can be formed.

The group I visited held all their classes in members' homes, keeping costs to a minimum, except where more space or special facilities were needed, such as for Art and Yoga classes. Some of their group leaders were experienced teachers -often retired after a lifetime of teaching children – but this was by no means essential.Knowledge of a subject and enthusiasm for sharing it was just as acceptable. They also organized visits to museums, concerts and art galleries from time to time, but each local group is autonomous, so the activities of one group may not be the same as another in a different area. The central office of U3A will be able to tell you if there is a group in your area, or even help you set one up if you have the energy and enthusiasm to do so.

This review of possibilities for study covers those that are most widely available, but it isn't exhaustive. The National Institute of Adult Continuing Education is an umbrella organization for organizations in this field, You may find other facilities in your local area, for example, regional arts centres, private teachers or educational trusts. Look in your local newspapers, Yellow Pages, noticeboards in adult education centres, in magazines covering your particular interests and ask other people who share those interests about classes they have enjoyed.

Finally, if you have a skill that you could share, you might consider teaching. People with specialised knowledge are always needed and if you have no teaching experience there are courses to help you acquire the relevant skills. If this is something that would appeal to you, approach your adult education centre, or U3A if there is a group in your area. Or organize a class in your own home or the village hall. There is great satisfaction to be found in sharing your skills and enthusiasms with others and some of the "youngest" older women I know are those who are doing that.

21

CHANGING CAREERS

THE SECOND HALF of your life is a good time to change career. You know your own abilities and interests, your strengths and weaknesses, whether you prefer to work alone or as part of a team and whether you like to be guided and supervised or would rather be your own boss. You know, also, that any work you embark on now is not going to be interrupted by pregnancies. You have experience and maturity to offer to any prospective employer, or to put to good use if you would rather work for yourself.

A surprising number of women do change careers in mid-life or later, often because the work they've been doing for twenty or more years no longer gives them any satisfaction. Their interests, desires and ambitions may have changed radically in that time, or they may have embarked in their teens or twenties on work that did not really interest them because they were unable to train for the work they really wanted to do.

Girls have always been more affected than boys by parental pressure to cut short their education and women who are reaching mid-life now are more likely than the generations that followed them to have been dissuaded or prevented from studying for a career, even if they grew up with brothers who were encouraged to succeed academically. Sometimes this would have been due to genuine financial hardship, or because there was no family tradition of higher education, but most often because of the notion that education was "wasted" on girls. The expectation was that a girl would get married within a few years of leaving school, that her husband would then support her financially and that she would devote the rest of her life to raising his children and providing for his comfort. Daughters of wealthy or aristocratic families were expected to make a "suitable" match, while those at the bottom of the social pile worked in shops or factories until they married (and often after, as well). Middle class more likely to go to university, music college, art school, etc., but even they were seldom expected to pursue a career in their chosen subject: it was taken for granted that they would put it aside on marriage.

Many social factors have combined to change this view of woman, but it's been a long time dying. The role of women in the 1914–1918 war, when they took on the work of men who had gone to fight, was a major turning point, and yet it did not make as much difference as it should have done to the lives of women after that war. They may have won the right to vote (at least, if they were over 30 – it took until 1928 for women to gain equal voting rights with men) but their educational, social and career status did not change very much. Most of the women who had been doing "men's jobs" for four years returned to domesticity when the war ended. Between the wars, less than 5% of women worked outside the home. Most professions were barred to them, and even many mundane jobs were closed to married women.

Their daughters' lives were not that different from their own, and even girls growing up after the second World War were often sent to shorthand-typing colleges or pushed into dead-end jobs when they'd rather have gone to university because "Mr. Right will come

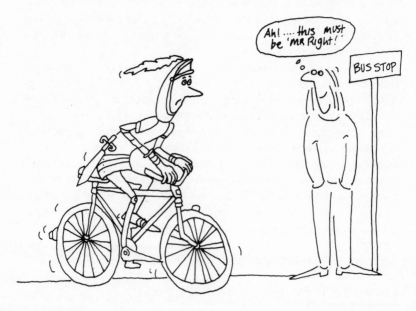

along before you know it". If they went on to any kind of higher education it was more likely to be teacher-training college, because teaching was a "womanly" occupation.

Those post-war teenagers are in their fifties and sixties now, and many of those who were frustrated in their original career ambitions have had the courage to return to them forty or more years later. And it can take more courage to make such a change than it would for younger women, because that generation were educated at a time when changing jobs, even within the same field of work, was seen as a sign of frivolity or instability.

Grace is 61 now: at 11 she won a scholarship to a girls' grammar school, where she did very well, especially at languages.

Her parents expressed pleasure at her exam results and her teachers expected her to go on to university.......until her last year.

When the time came to decide which university she would try for, her parents announced she would be going to secretarial college "So that you can earn a decent living".

"I was devastated. What I really wanted to do was to study in Paris at the Sorbonne, but we were much more in awe of our parents in those days, and of course we were legally 'infants' until we were 21. So I went to the very best secretarial college – it was more like a finishing school in some respects! – and as soon as I left I landed a plum job as a managing director's secretary, by-passing all the junior posts. My parents were delighted, of course. It justified their decision, but six months after my twentyfirst birthday I decided to go and work in France for a few years. They begged me not to, told me I'd regret it later, that having been lucky enough to get such a good job I ought to stay with it, and so forth. My mother sat me down and told me that skipping around like this would go very much against me when I applied for jobs in future – employers would think I was unreliable! But I went, anyway. With hindsight, I can see now that their attitude was entirely coloured by their own experience. My father had worked for the same employer ever since he left school, going back to his old job after five years in the Air Force. I some-times thought that his greatest ambition was to get a gold watch for fifty years' service!"

Grace worked as a secretary in France, had no difficulty find-ing work when she came back to England, married, had three children and did "nothing" (i.e., washing, cleaning, cooking, shopping, nappy-changing, nose-wiping, knitting, dressmaking, ferrying children to and from school) for a few years. At 40 she took a (very tough) course for professional interpreters and now runs her own agency offering translation and interpreting services.

A very large number of women who start new careers in mid-life are the ones who have spent many of their adult years bringing up children. Some of them resume careers that they broke off when expecting their first baby, while others want to do something entirely different, especially if the work they did before they had children was not what they wanted most to do.

Returning to a career you left twenty years ago can be quite challenging. You may find that techniques or outlooks have changed radically in the interim. You may find yourself working in a junior position under women younger than yourself. (Some firms will turn down older women applicants at interviews to avoid such a situation.)

Starting from the bottom in a completely new field may not be any easier: again, you may encounter prejudice against older beginners. Young bosses – whether male or female – can feel very uncomfortable about "junior" employees who are significantly older than themselves.

All the same, I haven't met one woman who regretted going back to work after a long break. Even those who found the going tough initially loved the mental stimulus, the excitement of doing something different and, often, the financial independence that their new careers gave them.

Many of the "second-career" women I've talked to have chosen to be self-employed. Not because this by-passes the problems of re-entering a career structure – it does, but it presents other, equally challenging, problems. The women who have chosen this path are often the ones with innovative ideas and creative skills that don't easily find a place in established businesses.

Sometimes these are the very skills that they've developed during their years of child-care and housekeeping. I've talked to women who have applied their cooking ability to outside catering, or their sewing skills to marketing baby-clothes, wedding dresses or handmade quilts, though unfortunately such "womanly" skills are often very poorly paid in relation to the time and effort involved. In order to make a decent living from doing anything that involves sewing or cooking, you really need to have a new and original slant and either a good grasp of business matters or a good adviser.

Paula is a keen knitter who has designed and made stylish and original sweaters for herself since she was in her teens. When her children were small she made all theirs, too, often with intricate patterns or personalized motifs. She started knitting for friends and asked very modest prices because "I enjoyed doing it. It's my hobby, so I didn't feel I needed to get paid a lot for doing it. But when my husband died I needed to earn a living, and realized that sweaters like mine were selling in smart shops at perhaps three times the prices I asked. Putting my prices up was difficult, because my friends were used to my old prices. So I advertised, found new clientele and charged a bit more. But when I counted the time I spent on each garment, I realised that I would have been better off cleaning!"

Paula sat down and brainstormed with a friend and worked out that what people really wanted were her original ideas and that it might be more profitable to sell knitwear designs than spend long hours making the garments herself."I produced a dozen patterns and advertised them in a craft magazine........no response! Then I realised the only way I was likely to sell my patterns was through wool shops. I had some success but not enough to live on, until I decided to open my own shop. I had inherited a little bit of money from my

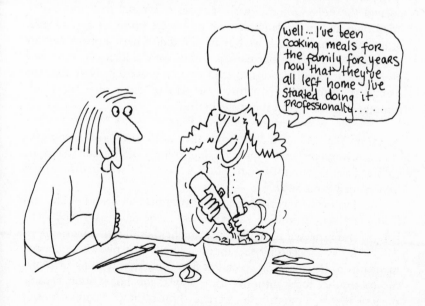

aunt so I used that as my capital, found suitable premises, bought a stock of yarns and opened up. Since then it has been marvellous. I enjoy my design work, I love meeting all the people who come into the shop and I make a good living."

I've quoted Paula at length because her story illustrates how it sometimes needs a bit of lateral thinking to turn your existing talents into a viable business.

Mary and Sue's experience was similar: Mary is 48, married with two adult children. Sue is two years younger, divorced with one son away at college. Mary had worked as an accounts assistant ever since she left school except for a few years when her children were tiny, and had come to hate it. Sue had not done any "outside" job since she married, but found herself needing to work after her divorce. Both of them are keen gardeners and they decided to advertise a gardening service called "Greenfingers". They got plenty of customers in their first summer, though the hourly rates were not good, but in the winter work almost came to a standstill.

"We spent that winter re-thinking and decided we had to offer something more specialized. Sue has a large garden fronting a road, so we planted part of it out as a formal herb garden, applied for planning permission to put up a small wooden building to use a shop and opened the next spring as herb specialists. We sell fresh cut herbs, dried ones and herb plants that we propagate ourselves and all sorts of herbal products which we buy in. We didn't have a penny to start with, but we talked to our bank and they were sufficiently impressed by Mary's accounting skills to lend us all we needed. Now that the garden is beginning to mature, we plan to do garden tours this summer with little talks about the herbs."

Some women turn to new areas of work through sheer necessity: like Paula and Sue above, they need to support themselves after a divorce or bereavement or, increasingly often, redundancy or enforced early retirement cuts short a career in which they would have happily continued.

Marjorie had worked in local government all her adult life, and held a very senior position when she was made redundant. She loved her job and expected to stay in the same field until retirement.

"I was shocked by the announcement that my whole department was to be closed down and at first I could only think of applying to another local authority for a similar job but it soon became obvious that other authorities were as short of funds as my own, and finding a comparable post was going to be well-nigh impossible. I had never thought of doing anything else and had no idea what to try, so I went to a firm of career consultants for help. The interview was fascinating, and helped me to see where else I could put my existing skills to use. Eventually I found a job in a concert-management agency. Anything less like local government you couldn't imagine. It is hectic, I don't earn quite as much as before and I love every minute of every day!"

At 50, Marjorie could have settled for early retirement and for some women that would seem like a dream come true: a reasonable pension and all the time in the world to study, travel, socialise or pursue hobbies. For Marjorie that prospect was less appealing than the excitement and involvement of an interesting job. There are no rights or wrongs attached to such choices, only finding the option that is right for you.

If you are already thinking about changing direction, you probably have a clear idea what you want to do next but if you are feeling restless, dissatisfied with your present work – or lack of it – but don't know else you could do, you'll need to think about your skills, interests and temperament and what kind of working environment would give you real satisfaction. Do you love being with people, or would that drive you crazy? Are your abilities intellectual or practical? Are you better at organizing or at making things?

You might try making a list of all the things you enjoy and all the things you are good at, to see if that suggests an area of work. Or bounce ideas off your best friend or, like Marjorie, consult a professional who can advise you. Be cautious, though, about career consultations based on a computer programme, unless it is backed up by plenty of commonsense and personal input: a very artistic, highly unconventional woman in her forties came out of such an interview with a computer print-out that listed "Marine Commando Officer" among the suggested occupations.

Well, Looking at our computer printout here, it seems that you'd make an excellent marine Commando..

Your choice of new direction may mean retraining, full time, part time, via distance-learning or any of the options discussed in the previous chapter. Many local education authorities offer "Returning to Work" courses for women who have not worked outside their homes for a long time.

If you opt for self-employment, do take advantage of the various schemes that exist to help people set up in business. If you have been unemployed, you may be able to get basic business training and a small weekly income for your first year in business through the Government's "Enterprise" scheme. Most banks offer help and advice on setting up in business as well as the financial backing that you may need. Don't be afraid of bank managers! They may be able to give you valuable advice. Your age is a positive advantage here: bank officials are more likely to consider your business plans seriously than those of a twenty year old.

If you want to change career, take heart from all the women who've done so before you and found enjoyment, satisfaction and independence.

22

ENJOYING YOUR CREATIVITY

ONE OF THE most rewarding prospects for older women is having time and energy to explore their creativity. Release from full-time child care or retirement from a job is often the point at which your imagination can be given full reign. Please don't think "Ah, but I'm not creative" and, please, never, NEVER, think "I'm too old".

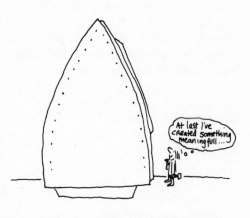

At last I've created something meaningfull....

Creativity is often thought of as a prerogative of youth: think how much fuss is made of prodigies. But perhaps that fuss is precisely because prodigies are the exception? The premature death of Mozart is far more newsworthy than Haydn composing great oratorios when he was nearly 70 or Richard Strauss, writing heart-melting songs at 84.

Of course, young people are creative: youth is a time of discovery and promise, but for the promise to be fulfilled, time is needed – time for exploration, development and deepening. Leonardo's early work would scarcely attract attention if we did not know the masterpieces of his maturity.

In an ideal scenario, the creative person is able to develop the skills of their craft alongside developing ideas and their own development as a person. For many creative women, though, the scenario is far from ideal: after a period of early promise the young girl may find herself blocked from the training she needs to develop her skills, for one or other of the reasons we have examined elsewhere in this book. Alternatively, she may get her training then come up against obstacles in the career field she has chosen or get started on a career and abandon it while she brings up children.

Such women often pick up the threads of their creative work in mid-life, when their domestic ties have loosened to some extent but they may find themselves struggling to express highly developed ideas with undeveloped skills. Rebecca's experience is typical:

"I married a fellow-student during my second year in art school intending, naturally, to finish my degree course, but I got pregnant within a few months and dropped out. We had two more children in the next four years and although I had tried to keep up my drawing after Rob was born the children needed all my time and energy. I can remember sitting in the kitchen crying one day because I hadn't painted anything for so long, and Mike saying that if I really wanted to paint, I would make time for it. He didn't understand that it was not something I could do in odd half-hours between the last feed and the next nappy-change.

I have to admit I wasn't miserable the whole time. Having babies is a different sort of creation, and I poured all my energy into being the best mother I could. There was a deep satisfaction in that but when Rob was about 17 I got depressed and knew that the only way out of the depression was to start painting again. It was very exciting to get started again but after that I found it absolutely frustrating having a mature woman's outlook and less technique than when I

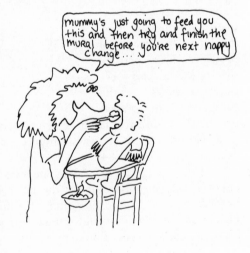

was 20. In the end, I went back to art school when Lisa, my youngest, was 18 just to polish up my skills."

I have chosen to include Rebecca's story out of a score or

more like it because she pinpoints two very important aspects of women's creativity.

The first is that giving birth is a supremely creative act. For many women, it is the most rewarding creative activity in their lives. This is not the same as saying that it is a woman's only role. Her ability to be a mother does not disqualify a woman from expressing herself in other ways as well but it often absorbs her totally during her fertile years. The advent of menopause brings, for many women, a shift of emphasis when their great store of creative energy finds other channels. It should not be a question of "either/or" but of "first that, now this".

The other point that emerges from Rebecca's account is that it is almost impossible to engage in serious creative work in short snatches. Florence Nightingale, once again, makes the pertinent comment "Can we fancy Michelangelo running up and putting a touch to his Sistine ceiling in "odd moments?" To achieve anything of worth needs consecutive, uninterrupted time and attention. So we see another reason why the different parts of a woman's creative life may need to follow each other consecutively rather than run concurrently. It feels appropriate and satisfying to a great many women to give their whole attention to their children while they are growing up. It can be just as right and satisfying to give undivided attention to other kinds of creation when the children become independent.

It is arguably easier for writers than for painters to start, or resume, work at mid-life or after because we use language all the time, but it is certainly no easier to write while bringing up a family than it is to paint. Mary Wesley, whose first novel was published when she was nearly 57 was not quite such a novice as the media would have us think, for she had been writing childrens' stories for years. Even to do this she had to retreat to her bed. There was no time for "serious" writing: "Of

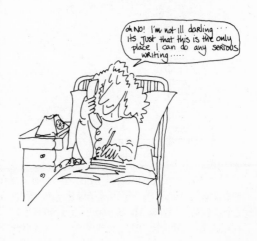

course, having children was a hindrance. When they were growing up there was no time for writing – and the husband was a block, too".

Minna Keal is a less celebrated late starter than Mary Wesley, perhaps because fewer people listen to symphonies than read novels.

As a young girl Minna entered the Royal Academy of Music, but left after one year because her father died and her relatives put pressure on her to help in the family business. Not until she was 60 was she able to pick up her interrupted studies. "I used my pension as a student grant" she said, and began to study composition privately. Her first symphony was performed at the Proms on her 70th birthday.

These women demonstrate that creativity does not wane with age. This is true even when considerable physical effort is needed to produce the end result. Georgia O'Keefe was still exhibiting paintings when she was 83, and we are not talking about genteel little watercolours! In 1965 when she was 77 she completed a massive, 8ft × 24 ft mural, the largest work she had ever undertaken. Martha Graham produced some of her greatest choreography in her sixties, dancing in much of it herself.

Lucie Rie, the potter didn't start working full-time until she was 47 and now, at 90 she is still potting.

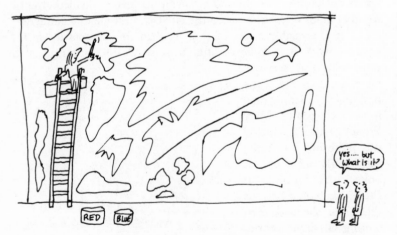

Not even physical infirmity can extinguish the creative fires. I think of Renoir in his 70s, his hands crippled by arthritis, painting on until his death with brushes strapped to his wrist, of Degas, almost blind and nearly 80, modelling clay when he could not see to paint any more. But, above all, because this is a book for and about women, I think of Elizabeth Frink.

She was working on a larger than life-sized horse when she found out that she had cancer. She had a few weeks to wait for an operation, so "I bashed the hell out of it, then I had my op. and it took me three months to get over it, then I came back and finished the horse." Her last commission was a 13ft high figure of the Risen Christ for Liverpool Cathedral. Until that time she had never employed a studio assistant, but for the Christ she found "a young man to lug buckets of plaster around" because she was physically frail and had lost a great deal of weight, but all the actual modelling of the statue was hers. A fortnight before the statue's unveiling, she was at the foundry, masked and goggled, putting the last touches to the finished bronze. She was 62 at the time. The Christ was unveiled on Easter Day 1993. One week later Elizabeth Frink died.

Up to this point, I have mostly drawn examples from the world of the arts. That's because it is the world I know best and which excites me most, but we find creative women in the sciences and medicine, women like Marie Curie and Elizabeth Garrett Anderson, for example, and among the great social innovators. And many of these women did, and are doing, their most important work from mid-life onwards. Emmeline Pankhurst was 45 when she founded the Women's Social and Political Union to fight for equal voting rights for women. In 1918, when she was 60, the right to vote was granted to women – but only those over 30 and it was not until 1928, the year of her death, that women gained equality of franchise with men. During those 25 years she went to prison 8 times.

I have also, I am aware, mostly written about "famous" women, which can give the false impression that "success" or the end-product are the purpose of creative activity. Nothing could be further from the truth. I have chosen to write about these women because their lives embody a truth that applies to all of us: that 40, or 50, or 60 or later is NOT too late to start doing what you want to do.

I hope, too, that their stories will not only inspire the thought "If she can do it, so can I" but also "If she found it impossible to use her creative talents fully when she was young, I needn't feel bad about the fact that I didn't, either". I have met so many women (and men, too) who feel that a major part of their lives were "wasted" because they were not doing then what they want to do now. Please believe that nothing you have ever done in your life is wasted. Every experience you have had is part of the person you are now.

Some women think that they have not been using their creative ability because so many of their skills are not recognised as "art". For thousands of years women have been making embroideries, tapestries, quilts, clothes, furnishings which are true works of art. If you have knitted, crocheted, sewn clothes for your children or decorated your home, you have been highly creative. Everyone who ever cooked a cake or planted a beautiful garden is a creator.

Yet there is another aspect to creativity, which has nothing to do with producing a cake or a sweater, a quilt or an oil painting, and that is the importance of doing something just for the joy of doing it. When I go to a dance workshop, I don't have anything to bring home with me...except a big grin! If you've ever sung in a choir, or spent a weekend making music – however humbly – with other enthusiasts, you will know exactly what I mean. There might be a performance at the end of it, but it is your experience of moving your body, using your voice or making music with friends that matters.

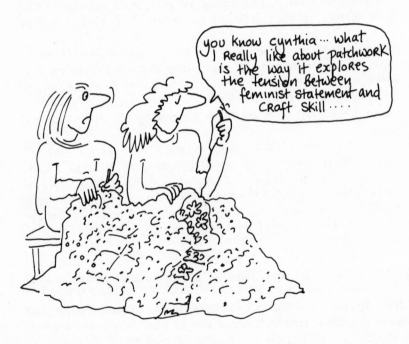

It's possible to approach painting in the same way. The summer before last I spent a week painting with a group of women – most of us over 40. Some of us were experienced painters,some had never held a brush before. It wasn't important, because we weren't there to "make art" we were there to paint for our own pleasure. We meditated and danced and painted, walked on the moors and painted some more. We laughed a lot and cried a bit and I came home with 24 pieces of painting – not one of which I would call "art". One woman made over 70 paintings in the same time. It didn't matter how much or how little we did, or what the end result looked like: what did matter was what each one of us experienced while we were doing it.

All over the country there are workshops and courses, classes and clubs where you can play with creative ideas. Whether you want to turn clay, make jewellery, arrange flowers, learn carpentry or welding, dance, sing, paint, spin, weave, sew, knit, crochet or play the double bass, there are other people who are doing it. You can find formal tuition or "fun" workshops depending on what you hope to get from the group.

You particular creative gifts may take other forms, such as healing, or story-telling, writing poetry or the history of your town or acting in the local drama group. You might fancy circle dancing or tap dancing or building your own house or a boat (to sail round the world?). Perhaps you would enjoy being part of a mural-painting team, or making costumes for the local carnival? Only you know whether you would most enjoy exercising your skills in private or as part of a group activity.

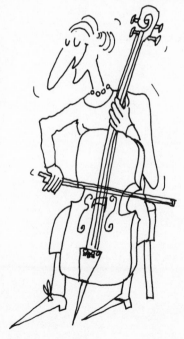

Whatever your choice, it will enrich your life. If you are like so many women at mid-life, you have probably spent years doing things for other people. Please give yourself the gift of doing something creative just for you.

FURTHER READING:
The Courage to Create   Rollo May   *Bantam*

23

GILDING THE LILY

THE GREAT THING about choosing clothes as you get older is that you don't have to follow any fashion dictates – though there's nothing to say that you shouldn't do so if that's what you would enjoy. You probably have a much clearer idea of what suits you, what you like, what you feel comfortable in than when you were a teenager so you can pick what you like from current fashions and ignore the rest. By "comfortable" I mean psychologically comfortable, as well as physically: if you are a countrywoman at heart you will probably feel "uncomfortable" in slick city clothes, even if they fit so well you are barely aware of them. You can create you own, unique style. You don't have to impress anybody or please anybody except yourself.

When you were very little, you wore what your parents chose for you. After that, possibly, a school uniform, and then whatever "uniform" your contemporaries had chosen to shock their elders!

After that brief period of rebellion, you may well have spent much of your life in clothes dictated by your role of secretary, mother, teacher, bank clerk or social worker.

Dressing just like all the people around you can be reassuring when you are young and unsure of yourself – that's why fashion trends have such a grip on teenagers – but by 40 or so, you probably feel much more self assured, so why not express that in what you wear?

Unfortunately, various conventions operate against doing so.

When I was 41 my 6 year old son told me that eye-shadow was "Not for your age". What made him think so? His best friends' Mummies didn't use eye-shadow. (I'm glad to say that 20 years later my son is totally non-agist.)

Then there was the incident of my sister and her jeans: she was also forty-something, and recently separated from her husband, when our father ordered, yes **ordered** her not to wear jeans while staying with him on holiday. He didn't even like his grandsons to wear jeans, but this particular pair of denims really enraged him because they had a designer's label on the back pocket which said "Easy". "I'm not having my daughter walking about labelled 'easy' on her backside" bellowed Dad! The fact that she was waiting for a divorce apparently made it worse, and he held forth at some length about "respectability" and not attracting attention to oneself.

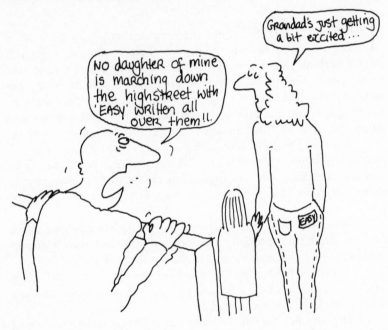

I recount these two little bits of family history because they illustrate how preconceptions about older women and their appearance get perpetuated. My father was born in 1906 and grew up when denim was only used for workmen's overalls, and "ladies" did not wear trousers. By the time I am writing about, he had come to accept that my stepmother wore shapeless corduroys to work in the garden or take the dogs for a muddy walk, but my sister's perfectly ordinary jeans really sparked off all his prejudices.

Why he should think he had the right to dictate what his adult daughter wore is another issue, but it also refers back to his youth and the social situation of that time, when very few would have questioned a man's right to impose his views about dress on all the women in his household: in other words, he had not really moved on from the "Victorian values" we looked at near the beginning of this book.

My young son's views about my eye-shadow were, to my mind, much more worrying, though not because of what he thought – when you are 6 it is very important that your Mummy should look as much as possible like all the other Mummies. What horrified me was that my contemporaries, in their late 30s and early 40s, had labelled THEMSELVES "too old" for a little discreet make-up.

Fortunately, times are changing and ideas, both about dress and the way men and women relate to each other, have become far less rigid but I still meet many women who have opted for a drab uniformity because they think that is what is expected of them.

"I'm 72 and I still enjoy clothes and cosmetics as much as I ever did" said Olive rather defensively. She didn't really need to say so because her clothes spoke for her: colourful, stylish and a complement to her personality. So why did Olive feel it necessary to make that comment, and why did she feel defensive? She'd been the butt of some comments about "mutton dressed as lamb", quite unfairly, for her clothes were in no way unsuited to a woman of her age. She wan't aping girls 50 years her junior: she looked exactly what she was – a well-dressed woman of 72.

Disapproval of older women who dress "young" goes right back to those discredited concepts "women's role is to have babies" and "women who don't have babies any more are not sexual". Once we accept that women beyond the menopause can have sexual impulses it becomes nonsense to censure them for wearing whatever they like. Even that presupposes, though, that the only reason for choosing particular clothes is to look sexually inviting. We need to acknowledge that it's alright to look good just for the sake of looking good.

The main difference between Olive's clothes and those of many of her contemporaries was colour and colour really does affect the way we feel. This has been well established by psychologists and colour-healing therapists. Operating theatres are painted green because the colour reduces stress, and even football clubs paint the visiting team's changing rooms pink because they hope it will make the make the visitors so relaxed that they won't put up much fight!

Exactly the same principles apply to clothes. I invite you to enjoy colour! After all, a mauve sweater need not cost any more than a beige one and, as Alison Lurie points out in "The Language of Clothes" "the gray shawl ... associated with the concept 'grandmother' is no better at keeping out drafts than a red or green shawl of the same construction".

Experiment with colours: what suited you 20 years ago may not necessarily be what does the most for you now, as your own colouring may have changed. You might have looked chic in black at 30, but at 50 it could make you look like one of the Addams family. Not necessarily: this is just an example. Some older women look stunning in black, and some women look dreadful in it whatever their age. But please don't feel that you have to retreat into darks and neutrals as a kind of middle-aged uniform. Go and try things on in shops, try your friends' clothes on, try your daughters' clothes on – you might be surprised!

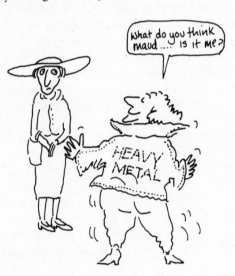

It's worth experimenting with make-up, too. In some large department stores you can try out different shades of cosmetics, and it doesn't cost anything. (They probably expect you to buy something, but there is nothing to say you have to.) Or you could book a session with a professional beautician. Why not have a "girlie" afternoon with two or three close friends, trying out each other's make-up, as well as the clothes? It could be the best fun you've had since your 'teens. (But do be honest about the results.)

If your hair is greying, grey or white, the balance between skin colour and hair colour will be different from what it was in your youth. If your hair was very dark the change will be particularly great, as it may now be lighter than your skin. For blondes and some redheads the change of balance is not so dramatic but the absence of yellow or red tones in your hair may mean that you can wear clothes in colours that didn't look good on you before.

If you really aren't sure what colours suit you, it may be worth consulting a colour analyst. There are several systems that help you discover what range of colours will suit you best. The most usual method is to sit you in front of a large mirror and drape you with lengths of different coloured fabrics, observing which bring out the natural colours of your skin and eyes in the most flattering way, and which drain you of colour. At the end, you will usually be given a booklet of colour samples covering the range that complements your natural beauty.

My friend Izzy (the same one who went rock-climbing) did this about 10 years ago: "I discovered that several colours I thought I could never wear actually suited me, and that the "safe" black I'd been skulking in for decades made my skin look pasty and dead. I won't pretend I went home and threw out all my black clothes at once – I couldn't afford to – but I gradually replaced them with lots of pinks and mauves and blues and I discovered that I felt better in them as well as looking nicer."

Clothes not only affect the way we feel about ourselves but tell other people a lot about how we feel. If we dress in colourless, anonymous clothes because we feel unsure about ourselves we not only perpetuate our bad feelings but signal to others that we lack self-confidence. Conversely, when we choose more colourful, or more shapely clothes we begin to feel better about many other aspects of our lives, too, and send out signals that say "this is a lively, interesting, confident person".

But, to quote Alison Lurie once more, "Thinking seriously about what we wear is like thinking seriously about what we say: it can only be done occasionally or we should find ourselves tongue-tied, unable to get dressed at all."

So........have fun!

FURTHER READING:

The Language of Clothes	Alison Lurie	*Bloomsbury*
Colour me Beautiful	Carole Jackson	*Piatkus*

24

CLAIMING YOUR PLACE IN SOCIETY

RIGHT FROM THE beginning of this book, we have seen that the attitude of any society towards older women influences the experience of the women in that society. If we want to enjoy the second half of our lives to the full, those of us who have reached or passed mid-life need to do whatever we can to challenge negative assumptions about menopause whenever we come across them.

Secrecy helps to perpetuate outdated ideas about menopause and the lives of older women because many of the prejudices are based on ignorance. So the first thing we need to do is talk: let people hear that menopausal and post-menopausal women are intelligent, active, sexy and fun! Let them know, too, that you have feelings and emotions: it is easy to forget that older people feel, and perhaps we have contributed to that by hiding our emotion at times.

Talk to younger women so that they know life does not end when their periods do. Especially if you have daughters, talk with them, because family myths about menopause are the most powerful ones.

Talk to other women of your own age. It can be both comforting and empowering to share your experiences. Talk to women older than yourself: there may be much you can learn from them.

Get active. Get involved. The more older women are seen to be doing things, the more this will come to be accepted as the norm. Getting active can mean whatever you want it to mean. For one woman it might be joining a theatre club instead of watching plays on television, for another it might mean driving the community mini-bus. My stepmother delivered meals on wheels until she was nearly 80 and most of her "clients" were younger than she was.

Another kind of active involvement is campaigning. If you feel strongly about any issue, do something about it. If you don't want to see a motorway cut through a stretch of ancient woodland, or a multi-story car park dwarfing the spire of your parish church don't just grumble. Write to local and national newspapers, organise a petition, write to your MP, make an appointment to talk to him in the constituency or lobby him at Westminster. Demonstrate in your High Street – and if nobody looks like organising a demo, perhaps you should be the one who does. Get together with other people: one woman alone may not be able to do much, but one woman galvanizing a group is a force to be reckoned with.

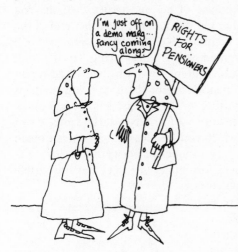

You may feel moved to campaign about issues that affect older women directly, such as the provision of adequate healthcare, pension rights or, conversely, the right to go on working. And don't forget that any any issue that affects women, affects all women irrespective of age.

I've met many women who would not have described themselves as "political", even previously shy and retiring women, taking such action over issues they felt strongly about. Sometimes these have been local issues, such as a hospital closure or toxic gasses from a waste tip and sometimes global ones, like the threat to the rainforest, or third-world famine. You may not be able to go off to the Amazon basis or a drought-hit area but you can get involved in fund-raising and spreading information nearer home.

I know one woman, sixtyish now and almost immobilised by arthritis who works tirelessly from her home to protect endangered animal species: another in her fifties who organizes her local group of Amnesty International. In fact, if you look at any national or international charity, you'll see how much older women contribute to the grass-roots organization. They do it because they care about the issues involved, and because they may have more time and energy to spare than women half their age.

You may be pouring that time and energy into study, or your

career – be it the first, the second or the fifth! – or an absorbing creative activity, and that helps to change society for the better too. Every older woman who goes back to school makes it easier for the next wave of mature students. Every time an older woman makes a success of her business, or shows her paintings in a small-town gallery, the people around her move one step nearer to accepting that age is less important than what the person is doing, or has done. At present, any "high-profile" activity by an older woman risks attracting attention simply because of her age rather than the real value of her achievement, rather like prodigies at the other end of the scale. Local newspapers love headlines like "Grandma learns to Fly"! Only when the majority of "grandmas" are busy flying, tap-dancing, pulling of major business deals or going away on their honeymoon will such things be regarded as normal. For the time being, perhaps we should welcome any reporting which at least lets readers know that older women are active members of society. All the same, if you see anything in a newspaper which you feel demeans an older woman by focusing on her grey hair, the number of her grandchildren, etc. rather than her real achievement, you might like to politely but firmly draw the editor's attention to that fact.

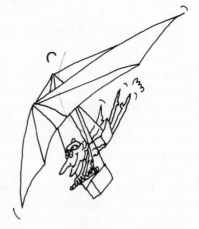

There are plenty of precedents for the older woman who is a valued member of her society. Many a mediaeval widow ran her late husband's estate and business, and that's without counting those who were a "power behind the throne". The Abbesses and Mothers Superior of convents all over Europe were responsible for large and sometimes very complex communities. Many of them were women of great intellectual or artistic ability as well.

In parts of India, post-menopausal women are able to come out of purdah and move about in society as freely as the men. They may become businesswomen in their own right and often take on the role of marriage brokers.

In some islands of the South Pacific, post-menopausal women were traditionally the sexual initiators of adolescent boys. While this is probably not a role must of us in the West would relish, it does at least recognise and honour the fact that women are still sexual beings after they have ceased to produce eggs.

The native American tradition honours the Grandmothers, as I have already mentioned. Perhaps I should add here that you do not have to have grandchildren to be a "Grandmother". All women who have come to the end of their fertile years are honoured for the knowledge that they have gathered during their lifetime. They are entrusted with teaching the ancient skills and traditions of their nation to the children and the Council of Grandmothers is respected as a source of great wisdom.

Older women have always been teachers, throughout the history of our race: we have passed on the healing skills, crafts and spiritual traditions that we received from our own mothers and grandmothers. We have handed down the family recipes, the songs and dances of our village and the tricks of the family trade.

These are things that we can all do. You don't have to have a qualification to teach your granddaughter to knit, or hand on your elderberry wine recipe to a younger neighbour. Do you remember the songs your grandmother sang? Or the special way your auntie made ice-cream? Can you recognise all the birds in your locality from their song? Whatever your skill, there will always be somebody who would like to learn it.

It may be that you have a store of precious memories. When Linda was a little girl her grandmother wrote her a series of letters about her own schooldays in Victorian London. She described the clothes she wore, the sweets she and her best friend bought on the way to school, the games they played, the escapades they got up to (granny wasn't afraid to let Linda know what a naughty little girl she had been!) Linda is a young grandmother herself now, and reads the treasured letters to her own granddaughter. You might like to set down some of your early memories, or write a narrative to accompany your family photograph album. In doing so, you'd be recording a little piece of history.

Being able to look both back and forward in time gives older women a more complete view of life, an ability to see events from a wider perspective. Janet, at 60, talks about her family: "Just within my own family I can compare the lives of six generations of women. I can remember my mother and aunties, of course, both my grand-mothers well and one of my great-grandmothers a little. Now I

watch my daughters living their lives and my granddaughters growing up. I feel as if a great deal of my life has been a struggle, and that
I am only just beginning to live the way I want to but I see my
daughters becoming women in their own right much younger and
my teenage granddaughters already self-confident and independent.
I'm happy about the progress women have made socially, though I
think there is a lot more to be done yet."

This kind of perspective can be really valuable to society –
perhaps another reason why menopause is an exclusively human
experience? Women from mid-life onwards bring their special
wisdom and experience to their work in education and medicine,
community and environmental work, charities, local politics and, of
course, their own families. There is not an area of life where older
women cannot contribute in some valuable way.

But the most powerful teaching you can offer is the way you
live your life. Live it fully. Enjoy yourself and be seen to enjoy yourself. Let people see that you are an independent, self-determining
woman. Our daughters and their daughters can only learn what the
life of an older woman is like by observing how we live. To be a
positive role model is perhaps the greatest gift you can give them.

FURTHER READING:

Growing Old Disgracefully	The Hen Co-op	*Piatkus*
Women of the 14th Moon	Ed. Taylor & Sumrall	*Crossing Press*

25

TIME TO GROW

O NE OF THE characteristics of living things is that they are able to grow. We spend the first part of our lives growing physically and mentally, we increase our height by inches each year, we learn all kinds of physical skills and how to behave in our family and in society. Then during our young adult life our personality develops along with our experience of life. Why should the next phase of our life be any different? In fact, the changes that we experience at mid-life can be a great impetus to further growth.

What you need is four hours of meditation or inner work per day!....

Change is most painful when we resist it most strongly, least so when we allow ourselves to move with it. I like the Taoist way of expressing this: "Don't push the river". Trying to push the river is a futile exercise, the water will always be stronger than you are. Far better to go with the current, not helplessly carried along, but swimming strongly and allowing the current to assist your progress.

One of the ways in which women try to "push the river" at menopause is denying that it is happening. The HRT/facelift/hair-dye response is one way of doing that. The woman who feels out of control, that she's going to grow older, sicker, weaker, less attractive, less wanted and there's nothing she can do about it, can be compared to somebody being helplessly washed downstream. Everything that I have put forward for your consideration in this book is intended to help you become the strong swimmer moving in harmony with the river of life.

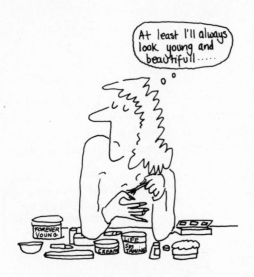

If we accept the changes that come about at mid-life, in our bodies, our relationships, our life circumstances we can use them as a basis for transformation. Do you know what really happens to a caterpillar when it is turning into a butterfly? I used to think it just had a nice long snooze while its wings grew but what really goes on inside the chrysalis is far more radical: the whole of the caterpillar's body breaks down into a sort of "soup" and provides the raw materials from which the butterfly will be made. I discovered this when I was going through some pretty big upheavals myself and adopted the butterfly emerging from its chrysalis as a symbol of my "new" self. When it felt as if my entire life was disintegrating, I would mutter grimly "caterpillar soup" and hope the wings were going to start sprouting before long. Remember that when you feel as if you are being turned inside out. Of course, you could opt to be a caterpillar for the rest of your life: it would certainly be less uncomfortable in the short term but think what you'd be missing.

Many women do, indeed, only start to fly in their mid-life years. Divorced women and widows often become more assertive – perhaps through sheer necessity – and discover strengths they never knew they had. Their new personalities may surprise their families and friends...and the surprises are not always welcomed! It can take a little time initially to get used to a strong, decisive individual if you've only known her before as "the wife of...", "the mother of...." or "so-and-so's secretary".

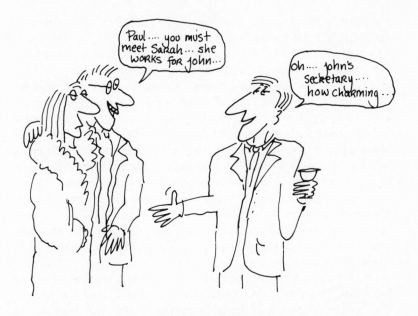

The process of becoming fully oneself was described by Jung as "Individuation" and some people enter therapy with the hope of discovering their fullest potential. Far more are goaded into therapy by the pain of their current situation and only later realise that they have grown as a person in the process. I have written in Chapter 19 about individual therapy as a way of dealing with emotional trauma but it is equally a powerful tool for personal growth.

Another approach is the workshop or group, of which there is such a huge variety on offer that it would be impossible to describe all of them. I can only say follow your instinct: if you see a workshop advertised that appeals to you, try it. One of the benefits of such group work is that you will meet people like yourself who are also spreading their wings, however tentatively. I sometimes think that the lunch and teabreaks when you can get to know the other participants are the most valuable part of any workshop! Some wonderful friendships have grown from such encounters.

Probably the most important aspect of personal growth workshops, though, is that they teach you techniques for self-transformation which you can use afterwards and, believe me, you do need to use them. No amount of workshops can replace time spent on inner work such as meditation, visualization and affirmation. If many of these concepts are new to you, you might find affirmations the most accessible of these methods to start with.

An affirmation is a positive statement which helps you change. For example, if you let other people push you around and you'd like that to stop, you might state "I am a strong woman who knows her own mind". Say this to yourself several times every day, and write it on a card to put where you will see it often: on your dressing table mirror, above your desk, on the door of the fridge, etc. I like to use coloured card and big letters in my best handwriting. If you enjoy looking at it, it will have greater impact. An affirmation is always in the present tense and contains only positive statements. "I will stop smoking tomorrow" is not an effective affirmation, because tomorrow never comes. "I do not need cigarettes" would be a more effective phrase. Once you understand the principles, you can write your own affirmations to help bring about whatever changes you would like in your life.

If you find it easy to think in pictures or imagine scenes and situations, you might find visualization a valuable tool for change. You might picture your body in perfect health, for example, or conjure up a scene in which you are effortlessly doing something that you currently find difficult. The more often you replay the successful scenario in your mind the easier it will become to bring about in real life.

For example, in my mid-fifties I started learning to drive and failed the test several times. Before the next test date, I tried visualizing myself driving the test route, doing all the manoeuvres easily, not feeling nervous, and – most important – being handed the pass certificate at the end! I did this first thing in the morning and before I went to sleep each night for two or three weeks, and passed the test without difficulty. This is a rather mundane example, which I have included just to illustrate how visualization works. You can use the same method to transform your life in far more profound ways.

If you imagine scenes in which you are interacting with other people, remember that YOUR inner work won't change them but it will change the way you relate to them and that, in itself, will often alter the response you get. This may sound suspiciously like day-dreaming, but it is daydreaming with a purpose, and it works.

"Thought precedes form" is the principle that underlies both affirmations and visualization. If you think about it, nothing has ever been made on Earth that was not thought about first: if you want to bake a cake you think first about what recipe you will use and which ingredients you need to buy, if you want to build a cathedral you will see it complete in your mind's eye before ever you draw up the plans or decide on what kind of stone to use. Exactly the same is true of your life.

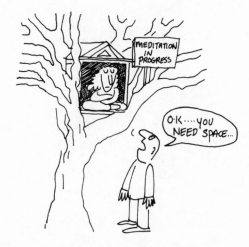

There are a myriad different ways to meditate, and some of them are virtually impossible to describe in writing: they really need to be taught on a one-to-one basis or in a small group. If you feel drawn to learn meditation, look around for teachers in your locality. I would, though, suggest that you try out more than one method and be very suspicious of teachers who insist that theirs is the only right way to meditate! No one way is right for everybody, nor even for the same person at different times. You need to find out which systems are best for you and you can only do so through experience.

For many people, working at personal growth brings them

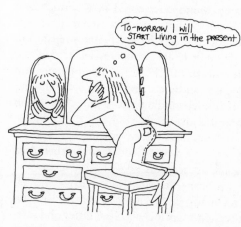

into closer contact with their Higher Self or spirituality. This has nothing to do with the notion of older women "getting religion". You can express your spirituality within the context of an established religion, or without any formal religion at all. One of the ways in which women have been focusing their spirituality has been re-connecting with ancient mysteries, especially those that concern

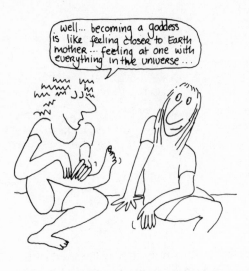

the Goddess. For one woman, this may mean feeling closer to the Earth Mother, or Gaia, and understanding our oneness with all her creatures, for another it may be exploring the myths of the Celts. The Celtic tradition has a powerful appeal for many European women who feel it is a way back to their roots, while for American women the Native American way often feels more appropriate (which is not to deny that many European women are drawn to Native American teachings).

When we develop our spiritual awareness, we come sooner or later to the consideration of death and our attitude towards it. For many women, menopause is the first point in their lives when they seriously confront the idea of dying, not because it is imminent but because the changes in our bodies make us realize our mortality. When you are young you feel immortal, even though you understand death as an intellectual concept. Menopause could be described as a little death, when one part of our bodies ceases forever to function. In fact, the experience of menopause can be a valuable preparation for dying. Once we know, through having experienced it, that the death of our ovaries is not the death of self, but a time of transition and that our life after menopause can be at least as rich and fulfilling as before, we have a way of understanding the greater transition which is the death of the physical body.

It may seem morbid to think about death in this way, but we can enjoy life more now if we are prepared for death, rather than fearing it. Conversely, living life as richly as possible now can make death easier to accept when it is near. Elisabeth Kubler-Ross who has worked with dying people for many years, observes that those who feel they have, in some way, wasted their life are often bitter and fearful. His Holiness the Dalai Lama teaches that resolving such issues as anger or hatred during our lifetime leaves the mind free so that we can die peacefully.

Mid-life is a good time for beginning to deal with those issues, for resolving any differences between yourself and the people in your life so that old hurts don't embitter you as you get older. It is a time for taking stock of what you have done and experienced up until now, and how you would like your life to be from now onwards – and then, of course, taking whatever action is needed to shape your life accordingly. It is a time for gently letting go of the young woman you were and joyfully embracing the mature woman you are.

FURTHER READING;

Affirmations	Stuart Wilde	*White Dove International*
Who Dies?	Stephen Levine	*Anchor Books*
Living Magically	Gill Edwards	*Piatkus*
Life Choices and Life Changes	D. Glauberman	*Aquarian Press*
What We May Be	Pietro Ferrucci	*Crucible*
Goddesses in Everywoman	Jean Shinoda Bole	*Harper & Row*
The Tibetan Book of Living and Dying	Sogyal Rimpoche	*Rider*
Older Than Time	Allegra Taylor	*Thorsons*
Mysteries of the Dark Moon	Demetra George	*Harper Collins*

26

WOW!

W.O.W.! MEANS "WONDERFUL OLD WOMEN"! A lot has been written about "Wise Women" and of course the wisdom of older women has given us so much. The human race would be the poorer without its matriarchs, priestesses, medicine women and teachers.

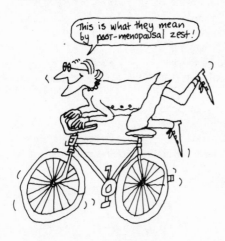

But wisdom is not the whole story. There is also what Margaret Meade, the great anthropologist, called "post-menopausal zest". By this she meant the energy and determination, the sheer enjoyment that older women often throw into all their activities. Margaret Meade was herself a supreme example of this, trekking around the world, living in primitive conditions while she studied non-industrialised societies at an age when she might have been tucked up safely in a retirement home.

Wonderful Old Women are not necessarily wise – at least not in any conventional sense. They may do things that the wise (or at least the sensible!) would shake their heads at.

I want to tell you about some of them, not so that you can look up to them in awe, but so that you can take inspiration from them.

Some of them are famous, some are unknown outside their immediate circle, but what they all have in common is that they have had the enthusiasm, the guts to do things they really wanted to do without regard to the dates on their birth certificates.

I am going to start with Dame Laura Knight, because she was my childhood hero. The first woman painter ever to be made a Dame of the British Empire, she had been pretty wonderful young woman, too, teaching art when she was 14, she went on painting right up to the time of her death at the age of 93.

Another Dame – Freya Stark, trekking in the Himalayas at 88.

Another childhood hero: Marie Rambert, pioneer of English ballet who was still turning cartwheels on her 80th birthday.

All the women I have written about earlier: Mary Wesley, still writing, Minna Keal, still composing, Lucie Rie, still potting, Marguerite Duras, still loving.

And who could fail to be inspired by Mother Teresa, continuing her great work of compassion despite advancing age and the failings of her own body.

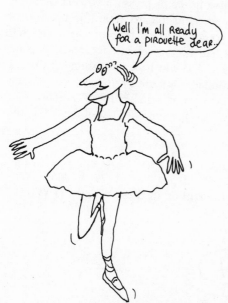

For every one of these celebrated women, there are thousands, no, hundreds of thousands of women, unknown beyond their immediate circle, who have lived, and are living life with courage and enthusiasm, making the world a better place just by being in it.

I have been inspired by so many of them: my own Grandmother, one of the first women journalists in England, who resumed her reporting career at 67; Ann who, in her 50's, gained both her MA and her City and Guilds plumbing certificate (in her "spare" time, between looking after her young son and her elderly mother);Julie who calls this phase of her life "me, no pause"; Shirley who at 65 rode on horseback from Spain to Scotland (that was nothing, really, she'd already sailed the Atlantic single-handed at 52); the Norwegian "Grandmothers Against the Bomb" who, at the height of the nuclear threat, stood in silent vigil outside the Parliament building in Oslo every Wednesday; Daphne who joined her first ballet class at 64, Miriam still going to art classes at 81.........

I'm sure that if you look around the women you know you will find just as many heart-warming examples.

But what I want to say most of all, what the whole of this book is really about, is that you, every single woman reading this book, are wonderful. You can take charge of your life, you can make sure that your physical body goes on serving you well, you can make of the second half of your life whatever you want, and you can do anything you decide to do.

So, is there something you have always wanted to do? Something you have never done before, or something you used to do but has been pushed out of your life by pressure of work or family commitments? A career you were unable to train for because of parental opposition, or that you abandoned to bring up your children? A hobby you have not had time to pursue for years? A place you have always longed to visit? Do you have an unfulfilled dream? Something crazy, unconventional, undignified, maybe even a bit dangerous? Something definitely "not suitable for a woman your age"! To fly a glider, write a novel, swim with a dolphin, visit the Amazon rainforest?

Do it now.

Because the most wonderful of all these Women is YOU.

WOW!

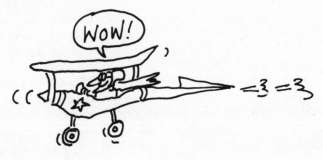

BIBLIOGRAPHY

Women of the 14th Moon	Ed. Taylor & Sumrall	*Crossing Press*
Growing old Disgracefully	The Hen Co-op	*Piatkus*
The Ageless Body	Chris Griscom	*Light Institute Press*
The Eat for Life Diet	Marshall & Heughan	*Vermilion*
Essential Supplements for Women	C. Reuben & J, Priestly	*Thorsons*
The Wright Diet	Celia Wright	*Grafton*
A Woman's Herbal	Kitty Campion	*Vermilion*
The New Holistic Herbal	David Hoffman	*Element*
Natural Healing in Gyneacology	Rina Nissim	*Pandora*
Menopause The Natural Way	Sadja Greenwood	*Optima*
Menopause	Llewellyn-Jones & Abraham	*Penguin*
Your Menopause	Myra Hunter	*Pandora*
The Amarant Book of	Gorman & Whitehead	*Pan*
Hormone Replacement Therapy	Gorman & Whitehead	*Pan*
Osteoporosis	Kathleen Mayes	*Thorsons*
Bone Loading	Simkin & Alayon	*Prion*
Yoga for Women	N. Phelan & M. Volin	*Arrow*
Bach Flower Remedies for Women	J. Howard	*C.W. Daniel*
Dictionary of the Bach Flower Remedies	T.W. Hyne-Jones	*C.W. Daniel*
The Healing Herbs of Edward Bach	J. & M. Barnard	*Healing Herbs*
Our Bodies Ourselves	Ed. Phillips & Rakusen	*Penguin*
The Language of Clothes	Alison Lurie	*Bloomsbury*
The Cause	Ray Strachey	*Virago*

APPENDIX A
ESSENTIAL OIL AND
HERBAL BLENDS

These formulae will alleviate symptoms for many women, but they do not replace professional advice. If your problem persists after trying these suggestions, or if you have any serious health condition, see your doctor, or a properly qualified alternative practitioner.

OIL QUALITY
Use the best quality essential oils you can find, preferably organically grown. There are many cheap ranges of oils on sale but they may be diluted, adulterated or otherwise of very poor quality and will not give the therapeutic results you expect from them.

Carrier oils should be cold-pressed. Hot-pressed oils are likely to contain a high level of free radicals, which can damage your skin just as much from outside as from within.

MASSAGE OILS
Essential oils are very concentrated and always need to be diluted before being used for massage. A safe and effective dilution is 3%, which you can make by adding 3 drops of essential oil to each 5 mls carrier oil. A carrier oil can be any good-quality vegetable oil, preferably cold-pressed. The most suitable ones are almond, grape-seed, safflower, sunflower and soya oils. Avocado and jojoba oils are good, nourishing carrier oils for face massage.

If you are using a blend of more than one essential oil, add 3 drops of the finished blend to 5 mls of carrier, NOT 3 drops of each oil. Some of the precious flower oils or "absolutes" such as Jasmine, Neroli and Rose, are even more concentrated and fewer drops are needed, so blends including any of these may add up to less than 3 drops per 5 mls.

5 mls is enough to do a face massage, 10 mls will do a back and for a whole body massage you will need 25–30 mls.

BATH OILS

Use 6 drops of essential oil to a full bath of water. Run the water, and when you are ready to get into the bath, add the essential oil and stir it about briefly. If you have a very sensitive or dry skin, mix the essential oil(s) with 10 mls of good quality vegetable oil first, then add to the bath.

HERBAL INFUSIONS

Using dried herbs, mix all the ingredients together. (If any of them are in large pieces, such as whole leaves, crush them first.)

Add 2 teaspoonsful of the final mixture to each cup of water and simmer for 15 minutes. Strain, then sip one cupful of the infusion three times a day. You can add a little honey if you like. If you make more than enough for one day's use, keep the infusion in a fridge and warm a cupful at a time as needed.

Here are some suggested blends for a variety of uses. Each essential oil blend is enough for one bath or one full-body massage unless otherwise stated. The herbal blends are given by proportion, so you can make up a large or small quantity as required.

ANTI-ANXIETY BLENDS
Massage oils:

Bergamot	3 drops	Camomile	7 drops
Neroli	6 drops	Lavender	6 drops
Ylang Ylang	6 drops	Ylang Ylang	2 drops
Carrier oil	25 mls.	Carrier oil	25 mls.

Bath oils:

*Bergamot	1 drop	Camomile	2 drops
Neroli	2 drops	Lavender	2 drops
Ylang Ylang	2 drops	Ylang Ylang	2 drops

*CAUTION: Undiluted Bergamot oil can cause dangerous burning when the skin is exposed to strong sunlight. Don't use it in the bath in sunny weather, OR add this blend to 10 mls of carrier oil before putting it in the bath. The dilution suggested in the massage blends is safe.

Herbal infusion:

Lemon Balm (Melissa officinalis)	3 parts
Passion Flower (Passiflora incarnata)	2 parts
Valerian (Valeriana officinalis)	1 part

ANTIDEPRESSANT BLENDS

Massage oils:

Bergamot	5 drops*	Bergamot	6 drops*
Geranium	5 drops	Rose	6 drops
Lavender	5 drops	Carrier oil	25 mls.
Carrier oil	25 mls.		

or

Bergamot	10 drops*	Clary Sage	6 drops*
Ylang Ylang	5 drops	Jasmine	6 drops
Carrier oil	25 mls.	Carrier oil	25 mls.

Bath oils:

Bergamot	2 drops*	Bergamot	4 drops*
Geranium	2 drops	Rose	2 drops
Lavender	2 drops		

or

Bergamot	4 drops*	Clary Sage	3 drops*
Ylang Ylang	2 drops	Jasmine	3 drops

*CAUTION: Don't use Clary Sage if you have had any alcohol or plan to do so within a few hours. Don't drive or use machinery after using Clary Sage – it makes some people very drowsy.

* Remember the warning about bergamot and sunlight, above.

Herbal infusions:

Lemon balm (Melissa officinalis)	2 parts
Lime flowers (Tilia europa)	1 part
Camomile (Anthemis nobilis)	1 part

This is a good blend if depression is making you jumpy and unable to sleep, but some people feel abnormally tired when they are depressed, in which case the following infusion would be better:

Kola (Cola vera)	2 parts
Rosemary (Rosmarinus officinalis)	1 part
Ginger (Zingiber officinalis)	2 parts

Don't drink this infusion too near bedtime.

APHRODISIAC BLENDS
Massage oils:

Black Pepper	1 drop	Black Pepper	1 drop
Patchouli	1 drop	Clary Sage	6 drops*
Rose	20 drops	Jasmine	15 drops
Carrier oil	50 mls.	Carrier oil	50 mls.
or			
Juniper	4 drops	Neroli	10 drops
Nutmeg	1 drop	Rose	10 drops
Sandalwood	25 drops	Ylang Ylang	5 drops
Carrier oil	50 mls.	Carrier oil	50 mls.

Each of these blends is enough to do two full massages.

Bath oils:

Patchouli	1 drop	Jasmine	4 drops
Rose	5 drops	Clary Sage	2 drops*
or			
Juniper	1 drop	Neroli	2 drops
Sandalwood	5 drops	Rose	2 drops
Ylang Ylang	2 drops		

* As always, be cautious when using Clary Sage – see above.

Herbal infusion:

Damiana (Turnera aphrodisiaca)	2 parts
Sarsparilla (Smilax officinalis)	1 part

BLENDS FOR FACIAL MASSAGE
For dry skin:

Jasmine	1 drop	Geranium	1 drop
Rose	2 drops	Rose	2 drops
Avocado oil	5 mls.	Peach kernel	5 mls.

For sensitive skin:

Blue Camomile	2 drops	Rose	3 drops
Rose	1 drop	Jojoba oil	5 mls.
Jojoba oil	5 mls.		

For crepey skin:

Frankincense	2 drops	Cypress	1 drop
Sandalwood	1 drop	Frankincense	2 drops
Avocado oil	5 mls.	Avocado oil	5 mls.

For wrinkles:

Frankincense	2 drops	Jasmine	2 drops
Jasmine	1 drop	Sandalwood	1 drop
Avocado oil	5 mls.	Peach kernel	5 mls.

CLEANSING BLENDS FOR FIBROIDS

Massage oils:

The following blends will help to improve lymph drainage as part of an overall treatment for fibroids. They do not, in themselves, constitute a treatment.

Geranium	8 drops	Black Pepper	2 drops
Rosemary	7 drops	Juniper	8 drops
Carrier oil	25 mls.	Pine	5 drops
		Carrier oil	25 mls.

Bath oils:

Geranium	3 drops	Juniper	4 drops
Rosemary	3 drops	Pine	2 drops

Herbal infusion:

Burdock (Arctium lappa)	2 parts
Cleavers (Galium aparine)	1 part
Echinacea (Echinacea angustifolia)	2 parts
Golden Seal (Hydrastis canadensis)	1 part
Sarsparilla (Smilax officinalis)	3 parts

BLENDS TO REDUCE HEAVY BLEEDING

Massage oils:

Cypress	8 drops	Cedarwood	5 drops
Frankincense	3 drops	Cypress	5 drops
Geranium	4 drops	Juniper	5 drops
Carrier oil	25 mls.	Carrier oil	25 mls.

Use either of these blends regularly as a preventive treatment. In an emergency, rub a FEW drops undiluted into the tummy.

Herbal infusion:

Beth Root (Trillium erectum)	2 parts
Periwinkle (Vinca major)	1 part

Drink 3 times a day in the week before your period is due and during the period if flow is heavy. If your periods have become very irregular, start taking the infusion when a period begins.

HORMONE BALANCING BLENDS

Massage oils:

Clary Sage	5 drops*	Geranium	10 drops
Geranium	10 drops	Parsley	2 drops
Carrier oil	25 mls.	Roman Camomile	2 drops
Sage	1 drop	Carrier Oil	25 mls.

* See the cautions above concerning Clary Sage.

Rub a few drops of either of these blends into your abdomen morning and evening each day. If there is anybody available to massage you, use these blends for massage occasionally. Don't use the same blend over a long period of time, but change from one to the other.

Bath oils:

Clary Sage	2 drops*	Geranium	3 drops
Geranium	4 drops	Roman Camomile	2 drops
Sage	1 drop		

*See the cautions above concerning Clary Sage.

Herbal infusion:

Chasteberry (Vitex agnus-castus)	2 parts
False Unicorn Root (Chamaelirium luteum)	1 part

BLENDS TO REDUCE HOT FLUSHES

Use the hormone balancing blends for massage, plus the following bath blends:

Morning bath:		Evening bath:	
Bergamot	2 drops	Bergamot	2 drops*
Cypress	4 drops	Blue Camomile	4 drops

Don't make the bath-water too hot.

Herbal infusion:

Use the same blend given above for Hormone Balancing.

BLENDS TO HELP IRREGULAR MENSTRUATION

In the early stages of menopause (perimenopause) the following blends should help to regularise the cycle. As menopause progresses, irregularity is a part of the normal process and is unlikely to be influenced by essential oil treatments.

Clary Sage	6 drops*
Cypress	6 drops
Geranium	6 drops

Carrier oil 30 mls.

*See the cautions above concerning Clary Sage.

Massage a little of this blend into the abdomen morning and evening for 10 days, beginning 4 days after the start of a period, then switch to the following blend for the next 14 days.

Bergamot	6 drops*
Juniper	6 drops
Pine	6 drops
Carrier oil	30 drops

If a period does not follow this course of treatment, discontinue the essential oils and start again after the next period.

Herbal infusion:
Use the same blend suggested above for hormone balancing.

BLENDS TO SUPPORT THE BODY DURING MENOPAUSE

Massage oils:

Morning blends:		Evening blends:	
Black Pepper	1 drop	Geranium	3 drops
Juniper	6 drops	Melissa	4 drops
Rosemary	8 drops	Rose	5 drops
or			
Cardamon	1 drop	Jasmine	10 drops
Geranium	7 drops	Myrrh	2 drops
Rosemary	7 drops	Carrier oil	25 mls.
Carrier oil	25 mls.		

These blends are meant to be used over a long period of time and must be alternated, as it is unwise to remain too long on any one blend. At any one time, alternate a morning blend and an evening blend, as they complement each other in effect, and use three or four times a week. Don't use them AT THE SAME TIME as blends given for specific symptoms, but they can safely be used in alternation with any of them.

Herbal infusion:

Chasteberry (Vitex agnus-castus)	3 parts
Wild Yam(Dioscorea villosa)	2 parts
Black Cohosh (Cimifuga racemosa)	1 part
Golden Seal (Hydrastis canadensis)	2 parts
Life Root (Senecio aureus)	1 part
Oats (Avena sativa)	1 part
St. John's Wort (hypericum perforatum)	1 part

Use this infusion regularly over several months.

BLENDS TO HELP VAGINAL DRYNESS

Use the bath, massage and herbal blends suggested for hormone balancing, plus the following:

Clary Sage   5 drops*
Geranium   5 drops
Sage   2 drops

Add these essential oils to 1 oz/30 gms of any pure, non-perfumed cream and mix thoroughly (Dr. Bach's Rescue Remedy Cream does very well.) Apply to the vagina daily for two to four weeks, reducing to three or four times a week after that. This is NOT intended as a lubricant to use during intercourse, but a long-term treatment, so apply at times when you are not likely to be making love.

The aphrodisiac blends (massage and bath oils and herbal infusion) are often helpful, too, at increasing secretion.

WHERE TO GET OILS AND HERBS

Some suppliers of good-quality esssential oils and herbs are listed in the next section.

FURTHER READING:

Aromatherapy, an A-Z	Patricia Davis	*C.W. Daniel*
Aromantics	Valerie Worwood	*Pan*
The New Holistic Herbal	D. Hoffmann	*Element*
A Woman's Herbal	Kitty Campion	*Vermillion*

APPENDIX B
SUPPLIERS OF ESSENTIAL
OILS AND HERBS

Aroma Vera,
3384 South Robertson Place,
Los Angeles,
CA 90034,
U.S.A.
High quality essential oils (some organic) floral waters and carrier
oils.

Fragrant Earth,
P.O. BOX 182,
TAUNTON,
Somerset, TA1 3SD.
High quality organic essential oils, carrier oils, base creams and
flower waters.

Ledet Oils,
P.O. BOX 2354,
Fair Oaks,
CA 95628,
U.S.A.
Pure essential oils, carrier oils, flower waters.

Neal's Yard Remedies,
5 Golden Cross,
Corn Market Street,
OXFORD SX1 3EU.
High quality essential oils (some organic), carrier oils, floral waters,
dried herbs and tinctures. Mail order from this address, also from
their shops.

Potters Ltd.,
Leyland Mill Lane,
WIGAN,
Lancs, WN1 2SB.
Dried herbs, tinctures, ointments, pills, etc., by mail order and through health food shops.

Swanfleet Organics,
The Swanfleet Centre,
93 Fortess Road,
LONDON, NW5 1AG.
Organic essential oils and carrier oils, etc.

APPENDIX C
RESOURCE DIRECTORY

1. WHERE TO FIND QUALIFIED PRACTITIONERS

These associations can give you the addresses of practitioners in your area with a recognised qualification. Please send a stamped, addressed envelope with any enquiry.

American Aromatherapy Association,
P.O. BOX 3679,
South Pasadena,
CA 91031,
U.S.A.

Association of Reflexologists,
27 Old Gloucester Street,
LONDON WC1N 3XX.

British and European Osteopathic Association,
6 Adele Road,
TEDDINGTON,
Middlesex.

British Herbal Medicine Association,
Field House.
Lye Hole Lane,
REDHILL,
Avon, BS18 7TB.

British Homeopathic Association,
27a Devonshire Street,
LONDON W1N 1RJ.

British Naturopathic and Osteopathic Association,
6 Netherhall Gardens,
LONDON NW3 5RR.

College of Osteopaths Practitioners' Association,
110 Thorkhill Road,
THAMES DITTON,
Surrey, KT7 OUW.

The Craniosacral Therapy Asociation,
c/o Sheila Kean,
3, Sandy Grove Cottages,
Horsley,
NAILSWORTH, Gloucestershire, GL6 OPS.

The Cranial Osteopathic Association,
478 Baker Street,
ENFIELD,
Middlesex, EN1 3QS.

International Federation of Aromatherapists,
Room 8, Department of Continuing Education,
The Royal Masonic Hospital,
Ravenscourt Park,
LONDON W6 OTN.

International Register of Oriental Medicine,
Green Hedges House,
Green Hedges Avenue,
EAST GRINSTEAD,
Sussex RH19 1DZ.

National Association for Holistic Aromatherapy,
P.O. Box 17622,
Boulder,
CO 80308-7622,
U.S.A.

National Federation of Spiritual Healers,
Church Street,
SUNBURY-ON-THAMES,
Middlesex TW16 6RG.

National Institute of Medical Herbalists,
9 Palace Gate,
EXETER,
Devon, EX1 1JA.

Register of Qualified Aromatherapists,
54a Gloucester Avenue,
LONDON NW1 8JD.

Register of Traditional Chinese Medicine,
19 Trinity Road,
LONDON N2 8JJ.

The Society of Homoeopaths,
2 Artizan Road,
NORTHAMPTON, NN1 4HU.

Society of Teachers of the Alexander Technique,
10 London House,
266 Fulham Road,
LONDON SW10 9EL.

Traditional Acupuncture Society,
1 The Ridgeway,
STRATFORD UPON AVON,
Warwickshire, CV37 9JL.

2. COUNSELLING AND THERAPY
These organisations can put you in touch with counsellors/therapists
in your area. Please enclose an s.a.e. when making enquiries.

Bereavement Counselling:
Contact your local Citizen's Advice Bureau, Social Services Depart-
ment or branches of CRUSE or MIND. In London, contact:
London Bereavement Projects Co-ordinating Group,
68 Chalton Street,
LONDON, NW1.

British Association of Art Therapists,
11a Richmond Road,
BRIGHTON,
Sussex BN2 3RL.

British Association of Counselling,
1 Regent Place,
RUGBY, CV21 2PJ.

CRUSE,
126 Sheen Road,
RICHMOND,
Surrey.

Institute of Psychosynthesis,
The Barn,
Nan Clarks Lane,
Mill Hill,
LONDON NW7 4HH.

MIND,
22 Harley Street,
LONDON W1N 2ED.

Psychosynthesis and Education Trust,
48 Guildford Street,
Stockwell,
LONDON SW8 2BU.

Relate,
Head Office,
Little Church Street,
RUGBY, CV21 3AP.

The Samaritans - see your local phone book.

3. STUDY

National Institute of Adult Continuing Education,
19b De Montfort Street,
LEICESTER, LE1 7GE.
Tel: 0533 551451.
Send s.a.e. for their free pamphlet "Learning When You Are Older".

National Extension College,
18 Brooklands Avenue,
CAMBRIDGE, CB2 2HN.
Tel: 0223 316644.

The Open University,
P.O. Box 625,
MILTON KEYNES, K11 1TY.
Tel: 0908 274066.

University of the Third Age (U3A),
National Office,
1 Stockwell Green,
LONDON, SW9 9JF.
Tel: 071 737 2541.

Women in Education,
The National Association,
P.O. Box 149,
PRESTON,
Lancs PR2 1HF.

4. ORGANISATIONS OFFERING WORKSHOPS

Benslow Music Trust,
Little Benslow Hills,
HITCHIN,
Herts, SG4 9RB.
Tel: 0462 459446.
Music courses of all types for students of all ages. Choir, orchestra, jazz, early music, etc., weekends and longer.

Centre for Active Therapies,
P.O. BOX 2299,
BARNET,
Herts, EN5 5PN.
Art, dance, movement, masks, etc.

Healing Voice,
Garden Flat,
9 Yonge Park,
LONDON N4 3NU.
Tel: 071 607 5819.
Voice workshops.

The Hen House,
Haverby Hall,
NORTH THORESBY,
Lincs. DN36 5QL.
Tel: 0472 840278.
Workshops for women only: writing, self development, assertiveness training, etc.

Life Planning,
77 Melrose Avenue,
LONDON, NW2 4LR.
Tel: 081 208 1996.
Workshops to help you assess your life so far and create a complete picture of your ideal future.

The Living Art Seminar,
11 Stowe Road,
LONDON, W12 8BQ.
Tel: 081 749 0874.
Art workshops, one day, weekend and longer.

Living Magically,
Hillcrest,
Duck Street,
CHILD OKEFORD,
Dorset, DT11 8ET.
A practical, fun-loving approach to making your dreams come true.

The Swanfleet Centre.
93 Fortess Road,
LONDON NW5 1AG.
Tel: 071 267 6717.
Wide range of classes and workshops: aromatherapy, art, dance, massage, voice, yoga, etc.

Women Unlimited,
79 Pathfield Road,
LONDON SW16 5PA.
Tel: 081 677 7503.
Wide variety of workshops for women: life changes, assertiveness, stress management, etc.

5. ARTS AND MEDIA

Campaign for Women in the Arts,
Great Georges Project,
The Blackie,
Great George Street,
LIVERPOOL, L1 5EW.
Tel: 051 709 5109.

The Network of Women Writers Association,
8 The Broadway,
WOKING, Surrey, GU21 5AP.

Society of Women Artists,
Briarwood House,
Church Hill,
Totland,
ISLE OF WIGHT, PO39 0EU.
Tel: 0983 753882

Society of Women Writers and Journalists,
110 Whitehall Road,
Chingford,
LONDON E44 6DW.
Tel: 081 529 0886.

Women Artists' Slide Library,
Fulham Palace,
Bishops Avenue,
LONDON SW6 6EA.
Tel: 071 731 7618.

Women's Media Resource Project,
89a Kingsland High Street,
LONDON E8 2PB.
Tel: 071 254 6536.
16-track sound studio, sound/film/video training.

6. INFORMATION AND ADVICE ON SPECIFIC ISSUES
Family Heart Association,
Wesley House,
7 High Street,
KIDLINGTON,
OXFORD, OX5 2DH.

Hysterectomy Support Network,
3 Lynne Close,
Green Street Green,
ORPINGTON,
Kent, BR6 6BS.
Tel: 081 856 3881.

Institute of Optimum Nutrition,
5 Jerdan Place,
LONDON SW6 1BE.
Tel: 071 385 8673

National Osteoporosis Society,
P.O. Box 10,
RADSTOCK,
BATH, BA3 3YB.
Tel: 0761 32472

Older Feminist Network,
c/o Astra,
54 Gordon Road,
LONDON, N3 1EP.
Tel: 081 346 1900.

Older Women's Project,
Manor Gardens Centre,
6-9 Manor Gardens,
LONDON N7 6LA.
Tel: 071 281 3485.
Advice on older women's campaigning.

Rights of Women,
52-54 Featherstone Street,
LONDON EC1.
Tel: 071 251 6576.
Legal research/resource/advice centre.

Women's Midlife Experience Centre,
318 Summer Lane,
BIRMINGHAM, B19 3RL.
Tel: 021 3359 3562 or 2113.

Women's Nutritional Advisory Service (PMT/Menopause),
P.O. Box 268,
HOVE,
E. Sussex, BN3 1RW.
Tel: 0273 771366.

INDEX

THE STORIES OF several women, famous and unknown, are quoted throughout the book. Rather than index them all by name, which would be meaningless to those who do not know them, the subjects they illustrate are all listed under 'inspiration'.